From navigating the spectrgen-
uinely crunchy household,   like
a chat with a wise (and fun   bout
detox; it's an invitation to infuse your days with authenticity, joy,
and a hint of delightful quirkiness.

GINNY YURICH, BESTSELLING AUTHOR; PODCAST
HOST; FOUNDER, 1000 HOURS OUTSIDE

Crunchilicious! Whether you've been crunchy for years or are
just crunch-curious, this book is for you. In *Really Very Crunchy*,
Emily shares a lovely approach to making your day-to-day life "A
Little Less Toxic."

SHAWNA HOLMAN, BESTSELLING AUTHOR, *A HEALTHIER
HOME*; FOUNDER, A LITTLE LESS TOXIC

Really Very Crunchy is a fun, authentic, and sincere book. An
absolute joy to read in a time when every human needs to read
it. We as a society have never been sicker. We have never been
more depressed. We have never been further from the values and
principles that solve both of these problems. *Really Very Crunchy*
couldn't be coming out at a more important and appropriate time.

TIM KENNEDY, *NEW YORK TIMES* BESTSELLING AUTHOR;
GREEN BERET; FREEDOM-LOVING AMERICAN

The book *every* crunchy mom needs to read. In a community
overwhelmed with tips on achieving optimal health in a sick
world, Emily manages to touch on the biggest (and even smallest)
health concerns—and delivers in a gentle, entertaining, nonjudg-
mental way. She's the crunchy friend we all need in our lives!

TAYLOR MORAN, CREATOR, LEAF & LEARN

Emily Morrow is a treasure! This benevolent and invaluable
book is filled with everything you need to walk the path of
natural living while also staying balanced and down to earth.

From recipes, stories, wildly inspiring knowledge, and practical insights, you won't want to put this marvelous book down. *Really Very Crunchy* offers a rich connectedness between those already living a barefoot-in-the-woods, crunchy lifestyle and those who are simply curious about it. Emily shares an unpretentious, intelligent, thoughtful, and humorous approach to natural living. Beautiful and inspiring!

JOHNNA HOLMGREN, CREATOR, @FoxMeetsBear

Really Very Crunchy

Really Very Crunchy

A Beginner's Guide to Removing Toxins from Your Life without Adding Them to Your Personality

Emily Morrow

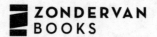

ZONDERVAN BOOKS

ZONDERVAN BOOKS

Really Very Crunchy
Copyright © 2024 by Emily Morrow

Published in Grand Rapids, Michigan, by Zondervan. Zondervan is a registered trademark
of The Zondervan Corporation, L.L.C., a wholly owned subsidiary of HarperCollins
Christian Publishing, Inc.

Requests for information should be addressed to customercare@harpercollins.com.

Zondervan titles may be purchased in bulk for educational, business, fundraising, or sales
promotional use. For information, please email SpecialMarkets@Zondervan.com.

ISBN 978-0-310-36752-9 (softcover)
ISBN 978-0-310-36754-3 (audio)
ISBN 978-0-310-36753-6 (ebook)

Any internet addresses (websites, blogs, etc.) and telephone numbers in this book are
offered as a resource. They are not intended in any way to be or imply an endorsement by
Zondervan, nor does Zondervan vouch for the content of these sites and numbers for the
life of this book.

The information in this book has been carefully researched by the author and is intended
to be a source of information only. Readers are urged to consult with their physicians or
other health professionals to address specific medical or other issues. The author and the
publisher assume no responsibility for any injuries suffered or damages incurred during or
as a result of the use or application of the information contained herein.

The author is represented by Tom Dean, Literary Agent with A Drop of Ink LLC,
www.adropofink.pub.

Cover design and photography: Micah Kandros
Interior design: Denise Froehlich

Printed in the United States of America

23 24 25 26 27 LBC 5 4 3 2 1

Contents

SECTION 4: *Crunchy Every Day*

Introduction

If you're reading this book, we've probably met on the internet. No, not like that, though I did have a Match.com account back in 2007. Unless you were one of the three profile views I got, you've likely seen me donning a linen apron, walking barefoot, and making light of trying to live my life in the most natural and organic way possible.

At the end of 2021 I was scribbling down aspirations I had for the coming year, and my list included things like "hone the skill of crafting pine needle baskets," "nurture a larger garden in the summer," and "select a suitable homeschool curriculum for my oldest child." I didn't even realize that my resolutions were all "crunchy." The pursuit of new abilities and talents rooted in nature was as much a part of me as the rhythm of my heart or the breath in my lungs. Cue the song "Just around the Riverbend" to get you into the spirit.

Creating a social media sketch comedy channel and posting a video every single day of the year was certainly *not* on my resolutions list. And I never expected to reach millions of followers or more than a billion views in a year. The seemingly sudden spike in chronic illnesses, autoimmune diseases, infertility, allergies, and learning delays is enough to make anyone question the conventional means of food, health care, and home products that are a part of our everyday lives. The natural lifestyle has been rising in popularity, and I happened to see the comedy of it.

When I started, the idea was to make videos about how the world perceived "the crunchy mom." In the early days of my content, I wrote a lot of sketches about how judgy crunchy people can be and how they can make you feel inadequate as a mom or as a person in general. A lot of the sketches came from my own feelings of inadequacy and being the one who was judged in those conversations. As you will see later in the book, I've had my fair share of run-ins with toxic crunchy moms, and they never leave you with a longing to be like them.

It was eye-opening to realize how many people, crunchy or not, resonated with the videos. This shared experience seemed to me a deep and profound one, transcending labels and stereotypes, and often had nothing to do with being crunchy. Everyone could relate to the feeling of someone talking down to you, making you feel like you will never make it to their level. And if you're not striving to make it to their level, then you're doing life wrong.

That's a horrible feeling.

And it led me to wonder, Why do people do that? Why do crunchy people do that? The answer came to me in a flash: No one wants to be wrong. The decisions we make for ourselves and our children matter! And if other people's decisions are counter to our decisions, then that means they aren't doing life right. Right?

As the channel grew, and when more and more people started to say, "Hey, maybe this lady actually is crunchy," I realized that the direction of the sketches needed to deviate some. It was getting to the point where my audience was trying to decide whether I was all in on making fun of and demonizing the crunchy lifestyle or, in a sly way, I meant what I was saying and believed that everyone who wasn't like me was doing life wrong. I was in danger of truly becoming a toxic crunchy mom—not just in a one-on-one conversation but to millions of people.

In this book, you will hear me say again and again that crunchy is a spectrum. There is no going all in, as there will always be compromises you have to make. I believe there are toxins in this world, both chemical and mental. In this book, I'll talk about some of those chemical toxins and easy ways to avoid them if that is your goal. But I also want to talk about the mental toxins. The relational toxins. I want you to realize that "crunchy" can be pursued without an air of superiority and actually should come from a place of humility.

I guess I'm trying to say that you can remove toxins from your life without adding them to your personality. This isn't a guide to being the ultimate crunchy mom you see in the videos—though I do like to stir the pot, so don't be too surprised when the really very crunchy side of me shines through. And it's not a guide to tell you all the decisions I make in my real life. I simply want to share what I know, put your mind at ease that not everything is going to kill you (at least not right away), and help empower you to make the best choices for your family.

Crunch-Level Quiz

Instructions: Select the answer that best represents your preferences or tendencies. Choose one answer for each question. At the end of the quiz, your results will reveal how "crunchy" you are!

1. **When it comes to food, I prefer:**
   a) Cooking whatever is in season and grown close to my home
   b) Cooking at home mostly, but Chick-fil-A is good too
   c) Whatever sounds good, but easy is king

2. **What is your attitude toward DIY projects?**
   a) I enjoy DIY projects and find them fulfilling
   b) I appreciate them but don't actively participate
   c) I prefer to buy ready-made products

3. **How do you feel about recycling or composting?**
   a) I'm passionate about it and do it regularly
   b) I do it occasionally but not always
   c) It's not a priority for me

4. **Which type of travel most appeals to you?**
   a) Camping in the wilderness
   b) Visiting a local farm or eco resort
   c) Exploring bustling cities

5. **Which words best describes your fashion choices?**
   a) Natural and earthy
   b) Comfortable and relaxed
   c) Trendy and sporty

6. **How do you feel about supporting local businesses and artisans?**
   a) I prioritize supporting local businesses and artisans
   b) I support them when convenient but not always
   c) It doesn't factor into my purchasing decisions

7. **When it comes to personal care products, I prefer:**
   a) Organic and homemade
   b) All-natural or plant-based products
   c) Popular and branded products

8. **Which activity would you choose for a relaxing evening?**
   a) Baking a loaf of sourdough
   b) Working on a favorite craft
   c) Watching a movie or TV series

9. **How often do you connect with nature?**
   a) Daily—I make it a priority to spend time outdoors
   b) A few times a week—whenever I get the chance
   c) Rarely—I prefer indoor activities

Now let's calculate your results and see how crunchy you are!

If you answered mostly a's, you're definitely crunchy. If you answered mostly b's, you are sort of crunchy, but you're flexible in your choices. If you answered mostly c's, you likely value ease and convenience, which take priority over crunchiness.

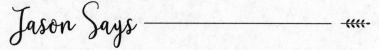

Jason Says

Hi there. I'm Emily's husband, Jason. I'm the one you see in her videos with the raised eyebrow anytime she presents me with some new crunchy idea. For some reason I've been asked to offer my take at the end of each chapter. If you're reading this, I'm not sure why you would want that, so feel free to skip ahead . . . or just read it. It's only about a paragraph or so. To get an idea of who I am, I'll share my results from Emily's Crunch-Level Quiz:

A: 1

B: 5

C: 3

It looks like I am decidedly *sort of crunchy*, though I mostly live "really very" crunchy because, well, look who I live with!

SECTION 1

The Meaning of Crunchy

CHAPTER 1

Crunchy Is a Spectrum

Picture this: I'm pushing the grocery cart down the produce aisle, looking side to side, not at the vegetables but to see if anyone is watching me. It's so embarrassing that my bell peppers didn't do well this year and I have to buy them. And what am I going to do when I get to the checkout? I forgot my reusable grocery bags, and I'm not sure this store carries paper bags anymore. Guess I'm skipping bags altogether.

My stomach drops when out of the corner of my eye I see Juniper's mom coming my way, organic cotton mesh produce bags dangling from her arm. I look down at my cart. There's no time to ditch the premade pasta sauce, but at least I'm able to hide the pineapple behind a mound of broccoli before she reaches me.

Sweat drips down the sides of my face, which reminds me I need to buy more limes for deodorant.

Our eyes meet. Then I remember the mayonnaise in my cart. They were out of the avocado oil kind. I push the cart away from me.

"Goodness, I can't believe people would just abandon their carts in the middle of the produce aisle like this! How are you doing? Haven't seen you in a long time. I'm just here to find some lemons. Doing a liver detox this week. Can't have enough!"

If there is one question I get more often than others, it's some variation of "Wait, are you crunchy in real life?" or "Is this satire, or is this real?" If it isn't obvious by this point, the truth is, I *am* a crunchy mom. There. I said it. The truth is out. But to me, that doesn't quite answer the question because there is one critical distinction between the real Emily (the one writing this book) and the Emily you see online, and that's the ability to adapt. Many of the comedic situations you see in my online skits come from real situations in my life, but the online Emily portrays what I'd be like in those situations if I were unrelenting, completely unwavering in my convictions as a crunchy mom.

When I'm asked whether I'm actually crunchy, I don't often give a straight answer. To say yes or no would be to solidify in their minds who I am and that the character I have created for social media is either 100 percent me or 0 percent me.

I am passionate about making healthy choices, so it is me but dialed up from about a six or seven to a ten or eleven, with an added splash of snark or judgment for comedy's sake. No, I didn't start a zero-waste tree removal company where

I communicate with beavers in their own language. Yes, I do like to go barefoot when I can. Do I make our guests sleep on the floor because of the numerous benefits? No. Would I bring sauerkraut to a movie theater? Maybe . . .

Most importantly, no, I don't judge anyone for the choices they make for their family. I don't know your life, just like you don't know mine. I assume everyone is trying their best. Maybe you're not crunchy like I am. Maybe you're more crunchy! Maybe you're wondering what *crunchy* even means. That's an important piece of information before we continue this book.

The term originated in the 1960s and '70s with the hippie, earth-loving crowd because they were known for the crunchy granola they ate—like, actually crunchy. The term stuck, and these days the people who identify as "crunchy" or "granola" range from people who do a lot of hiking and camping to people who exclusively homeschool to people from all walks of life who focus on a holistic approach to achieving good health and wellness. Crunchy people have some awareness of their impact on the environment and love to throw around words like *sustainable* and *counterculture*. Once someone questions what kind of additives are in foods and how chemicals added to products might be affecting their body, they are at least slightly crunchy. Crunchy is a spectrum, and we're all different degrees of crunchiness.

Crunchy isn't a singular group of people. It's not a clique. It's not an organized community any more than a group of soccer moms or friends who get together on Fridays for game night. Sure, crunchy people may hang out in groups, but that's often because they're researching the same kinds of things in the pursuit of trying to make their lives healthier. You don't learn how to make homemade marshmallows from beef gelatin by accident, after all.

The term *crunchy* might feel divisive or holier-than-thou, which is honestly where my parody account came from—I started my journey at ground zero like the average person, and it was intimidating to find my way! Nowadays, I look at the term as lighthearted and even funny. It's a quick way to describe someone who's trying to get as close to the natural way of living as our modern world allows.

Here is the truth as I've learned it: a crunchy life needs to be all about balance. An unbalanced approach to life isn't usually a happy one, no matter what the situation is.

Thinking in extremes might be more natural (get it?), but I find that trying to maintain that sort of rigid control only leads to feelings of guilt and shame. Guilt and shame can creep up in many ways. There's the kind of guilt that comes with "I'm not doing enough," and there's the kind of guilt that comes with "Oh, man, I messed up . . ." Those are two things we need to get rid of right off the bat.

It's easy to feel like you're not doing enough, especially when you're following a bunch of crunchy homesteader accounts on Instagram. But we must remember that everyone is on a journey, and part of what we're learning is what our limits are. Oh, and we also must remember not to compare ourselves with crunchy homesteader people on Instagram. Trust me, it's a losing battle for most of us.

There's danger beyond the social media comparison game too. I think the internet is both the best and worst thing that has happened to our society. When it comes to learning, it can be the best. But what if what you're learning isn't true? We can't know how much that beautiful crunchy homesteader was paid to sell a product, so is that account a source of solid information? Do you trust the studies funded by large companies that have a vested interest in the positive or negative outcomes of those studies? Or do you trust Juniper's mom on Reddit who said she did the opposite of the study's conclusion and it changed her life for the better?

Every single topic you research, especially relating to health, can lead you down some weird rabbit holes. If you're not careful, you'll eventually find yourself in a place that has absolutely nothing to do with what you were originally trying to research. There's a guy in this corner of the internet who says the carnivore diet is the best—eat like a caveman and see the results. There's a gal in that corner of the internet who's a vegetarian and says life couldn't be better! Oh, and don't forget about that whole thread dedicated to how the government is trying to control your mind through tap water.

I know, right? It's enough to make your head spin and cause that guilt and shame to creep in, but now with an added bonus: *panic*. What's a wannabe crunchy person to do? The new information from the rabbit hole (true or not) may cause you to question your situation and may even cause anxiety. You have to ask yourself: Is the anxiety this information is causing worse for me than not implementing the changes the information suggests? In other words: Am I healthier if I'm not worried about all these things?

The answer to this predicament is balance.

We need balance because, according to anywhere you look on the internet, *everything* is trying to kill you.

I envy people who were adults before the twenty-four-hour news cycle came to be. I think it started the need to have the latest information *right now,* which then leads to rushed information and opinions counting as "news." And the internet is no different. People want to be relevant. Companies want to make money, so they will write an article about anything, all with the goal of getting more clicks so they can sell you ads. And no, that's not a conspiracy theory; that's just how business works.

But people didn't used to live in fear all the time. I don't think the information age we are living in is inherently bad, as it has also done a lot of good for people, but I've known many people (myself included) who have felt crippled by too much information, with a lot of that information being conflicting.

If you're "going on a crunchy journey," then I suggest starting with small decisions. From there, you can open yourself up for more as you see fit. And if things start to make you worry or if you can't sleep at night because of what you're reading, then it's time to take a step back. You know what's worse than drinking a glass of tap water? Staying up all night worrying about drinking a glass of tap water!

The answer *has to be* balance. Reframe the panic to favor balance whenever you can. Ask yourself: What do I already know? What is the best choice I can make for my family with the information and resources available to me?

Which is better: eggs or pastries? Nutritionally, eggs win here, but that doesn't mean you're doing something wrong if you and your kids buy or make some pastries to enjoy some Saturday morning. Are you in France? If so, you'd better be choosing pastries.

Which is better: 100 percent wool or polyester? Wool takes the trophy, as wearing polyester all the time can be problematic. But take it from me, a wool bathing suit is pretty itchy.

Which is better: sitting in front of a screen or hiking in the woods? Personally, I think hiking always wins here. But there are some great documentaries worth watching. (See? Balance!)

Which is better: drinking filtered water or drinking straight from the sink? Don't die of thirst just because filtered water isn't an option!

Which is better: going out to eat with friends or staying home because the food they're eating at the restaurant isn't organic? My husband, Jason, and I have learned to prioritize our community over our organic preferences, and I'm never disappointed by that choice.

Crunchy is a spectrum. It's not a level or award you achieve. You don't get a fancy pink Cadillac once you've gained a certain number of crunchy points (a Cadillac wouldn't be crunchy, anyway. It would need to be a Subaru or, better yet, a bicycle). Crunchy shouldn't be scary or exclusive; it's just a fun way to describe someone who is making healthier, more natural choices. My goal is to help you see that being crunchy is much more accessible than you previously thought—maybe you're already crunchy and you don't even know it!

I hope you've realized by now that this book isn't about making you crunchy or saying you need to be crunchy. If anything, my aim is that you'll come away from reading it with the outlook of discovering yourself. I want you to find out who *you* are. Do what you think is best for *your family*. Can you go further, deeper, in your crunchy journey? Everyone can! I mean . . . except for me. I am, after all, really very crunchy.

What's your favorite go-to snack?

SILKY	SCRUNCHY	REALLY VERY CRUNCHY
Individually wrapped HoHos	Kirkland trail mix	Foraged berries

Jason Says ───────────────── ◄◄◄

I'm just gonna say it. Oreos are better than just about any cookie out there. Yeah, I know they are made in a lab and are probably just as akin to laundry detergent as they are to actual cookies, but you will never convince me they aren't fantastic. But being crunchy is about small choices, right? If you're at a party, and you find a tray with Oreos on them, what would be the crunchy decision to make? Easy. You eat only eight of them instead of the twelve you would have eaten. Crunchy decision achieved. But seriously, I think what Emily is getting at here might be that if you're going to have Oreos, how about you only eat a few when you're at a party. Maybe forgo adding them to your shopping cart next time you're at the grocery store so they aren't sitting half-open on the kitchen counter. Who am I kidding? They would be gone before I got home.

CHAPTER 2

Don't Be Toxic

"This is actually so toxic."

That's a response I never expected to receive in reply to a birthday gift. I mean, I knew my budget was only ten dollars, but I thought some top-shelf grocery store hand soap and a tea towel were pretty safe choices. I had that very hand soap tucked under my bathroom cabinet to pull out as my fancy soap when guests came over.

I looked around the room, stunned. What do you even say to that?

I finally mumbled a meager, "Oh, maybe you can just regift it?"

To which Amy replied, "I would never knowingly give someone toxins."

I have never felt so small in my adult life. Here I was, trying to make a friend (a lifetime struggle of mine), and I gave her poison! Poison disguised as a lemon verbena–scented hand soap made with olive oil and aloe vera. I was so embarrassed.

As we were leaving the get-together, Amy told me my gift was a "nice thought" and that I should consider getting an app that could tell me on a scale of zero to ten how toxic products are so I could make sure I was getting the cleanest products possible (zero being the least toxic and ten being the absolute worst!). Wasn't the very purpose of soap to be clean? I downloaded the app as soon as I got in the car. My hands shook as I typed in the brand name of the soap I had purchased, followed by "lemon verbena" to see how toxic this cleansing agent really was. A little hand soap emoji blinked on the screen, taunting me while the app retrieved my results.

An eight. I'd given someone an *eight*! Should I follow her home and apologize? Should I call everyone who had washed their hands in my home in the last thirty days and let them know they had been exposed to an eight-out-of-ten toxic substance? If the Chernobyl disaster was a ten out of ten on the scale of toxicity, how was it even legal to sell an eight-out-of-ten product? I was pregnant at the time, and I had definitely used the guest hand soap. *Would my baby be okay?*

If this soap was so toxic, what else in my home was killing me slowly? I'd used a Swiffer WetJet to mop my floors that morning. Was that okay? What about my dish soap? I used that on stuff I ate from! What about Windex glass cleaner? I was pretty sure I'd accidentally inhaled some of that. Was it only cleaning supplies? What about shampoo and conditioner? Body soap? Why wouldn't the bottle come with a warning?

I didn't understand why one of the nicest people I knew made me feel so small. As I've continued my journey, I have thought about this exchange a lot and realized it's good to try your best to be unoffendable and also try not to offend. It's best to meet people where they are and try to understand where they're coming from, whether you're the one giving the toxic hand soap or the one receiving it. Sometimes I wonder whom I may have done this to without thinking about it. Whom have I looked directly in the eyes and said, "This is so toxic!" assuming we were on the same page when we actually weren't? Having been on both sides of this type of interaction, I can see how important it is to assume the best in people, be quick to forgive, and know that most people aren't out to tear you down. Amy probably should've opened the gift and just said, "Thanks!"

Our world is full of toxins; this is not new information. Our bodies were created to be able to filter out and detox most of what the natural world has to throw at us. But now we are exposed to more and more toxins through things like hand soap and glass cleaner and candles and shampoo and so on. Because of this, our toxic load is heavier than it has ever been, and when we aren't able to detox at the alarming rate we are being exposed to toxins, our bodies respond in different ways. Many people have found their way to the crunchy life because they're trying to feel better.

For anyone already on a crunchy journey, it can be tempting to spew facts. And people are naturally curious, so don't worry, there will be plenty of opportunities to share information you're passionate about. But this should be done in the proper time and place. Vikkie was someone who handled my ignorance with grace. Our first encounter involved me offering her and each of her three beautiful children a slice of rainbow cake. Yes, it is what it sounds like: a cake pumped full of every color of food dye imaginable for the sake of looking pretty. The icing on the outside is white, so you think you're about to get a plain piece of cake, then you cut it open and, *bam*, you're shocked and delighted to see a spectrum of colors. Such a fun cake! Vikkie just smiled and said, "No thanks." Later, with a gentle demeanor, she told me there's a lot of evidence that food dye isn't great for your health and that it's linked to a bunch of different behavioral problems in children—some dyes are even known carcinogens. Many of the common dyes used in the US are banned in European countries. She didn't mention the rainbow cake. I was grateful.

As mortifying as the great soap blunder of 2017 was, my crunchy journey started before she called me out. My husband and I were living in a van down by the river. Well, it was actually a lake, and it was a 1994 Damon Challenger RV complete with teal shag carpet and baby-blue velvet-covered valances. How did we get there and *why would I admit such a thing?*

My husband, Jason, and I met in college while I was waiting for an elevator. I was holding a bottle of V8 V-Fusion juice; it couldn't have been that bad, right? It's V8!

"Is that for your car?" he asked, pointing to the juice. That may have been the lamest, cheesiest joke I'd ever heard, but at that moment, I knew he was the one. After we graduated, we got married and decided we wanted to live an adventurous life, so we left everyone we knew and moved to the first place to offer him a job: Jesup, Georgia. A quaint classic Southern town of ten thousand, home to the sweetest people in the world, a paper mill, and not much else. With not much to do, we often found ourselves bicycling to the Dairy Queen for a Pecan Mudslide, justifying the one-mile bike ride as enough to cancel out the calories from the ice cream.

At this point in my journey, I was what you would call silky. What's silky, you ask? It's pumpkin spice–scented candles in the fall. It's saying yes to the lollipop at the bank when the clerk asks if your kid can have one. It's a go-with-the-flow, whatever's-convenient, carefree kind of attitude. It is the very definition of (and I'm saying this in the least-Amy way possible) "ignorance is bliss." Silky is the exact opposite of crunchy.

After three months of small-town living, we decided it was time for a grander adventure, so we packed up our things and moved to South Korea to teach English as a second language (ESL) to elementary students. Not everyone was as gung ho about us moving so far away. Our friends and family showed a lot of concern about the aggressive speeches made by the North Korean leader, which seemed to dominate the news a couple of times every year. In general, the South Korean citizens didn't seem worried about it, so we weren't either.

South Korea is where I was introduced to fermented foods and things that *seemed* healthy because they *tasted* healthy. I'm an adventurous eater and enjoyed trying a lot of new dishes. Back then I thought eating chicken feet was outrageous, while future me has a steady supply of chicken feet to add to bone broths for the extra collagen. I'd like to say we stuck with eating traditional Korean foods, but my husband and I were most excited about gas station cheesy ramen and entire restaurants devoted to different types of toast. Oh, and in a time before DoorDash and Grubhub, we could order McDonald's to be delivered to our apartment in under twenty minutes. It was magical.

A theme in our relationship has been to always say yes to opportunities. I know it sounds cliché, like we're trying to live out the *Yes Man* Jim Carrey rom-com of the late 2000s, but it had served us well so far. ESL employment contracts in Korea typically last one year, and after two years there we were itching to travel more. We took the money we saved to pay off our student loans and instead spent most of it to travel around Europe. Dave Ramsey would be ashamed. I have no regrets, but Dave and I can both agree that you really should give up Starbucks, even if we have different reasons.

After several months of galivanting around Europe, we moved back to America to try to figure out what we should do with ourselves. We tried our hand at a few odd jobs, and that's when the opportunity arose to sell all our possessions and move into an RV and travel full time. Of course we said yes! My husband had self-published a few novels that were making just enough money for us to live on as long as we "park hosted" to get our camping spot for free, filled up our gas tank only every couple of months, and drove a scooter as our main form of transportation.

This was in 2013 before full-time RV living was a popular trend among young couples, so every park where we applied to be park hosts was ecstatic because they could utilize our youth for some jobs that required manual labor. Among other full-timers we were universally known as "the kids." We were having the time of our lives, but one month, my husband's royalties were pretty low, and that's when my crunchy journey began. I frantically googled "easy ways to save money on groceries without being a crazy coupon lady" and found an article that suggested you only buy food that has five ingredients or less. (Side note: Frantic googling is a surefire sign of crunchiness.) I had never paid much attention to food labels except to look at calories, so when I started counting the ingredients, that cut out a lot of options. Once we started eating whole foods and some processed foods with fewer, simpler ingredients, we not only saved money, but we also started to feel better. Things we thought were normal, like heartburn, constipation, bloating, and headaches, all seemed to disappear. We both had more clarity of mind and more energy, which we needed for shoveling fifty fire pits and cleaning campground bathrooms.

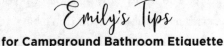

for Campground Bathroom Etiquette

1. Treat others' toilets the way you want yours to be treated.
2. The bathrooms are not a kennel for your dog named Root Beer—Jason's butt still has a scar from that bite.
3. The carcass from your hog roast does not belong in the bathroom trash can.
4. If you open a window, close it, because someone has to get out all the birds, bats, squirrels, and spiders that sneak in.

Using a small scooter as your only form of transportation presents some interesting situations. Like when we stayed in Gulf Shores in January and there was a rare giant ice storm. Remember the *Dumb and Dumber* freezing-scooter scene? Yeah, that was us, right down to me wearing a bicycle helmet instead of a motorcycle helmet because that's what we had. (Is it awkward that I keep comparing my life to Jim Carrey comedies?) Or there was the time we were park hosting at Prairie Creek Redwoods State Park in California. It was stunning. There was no internet access there, and the only grocery store was in the post office. The groceries were incredibly expensive, and all the food had way more than five ingredients. So we did what any sane people would do: we rode our scooter forty miles on the shoulder of the highway to get to the nearest grocery store. You know how you load up your arms with as many groceries as possible so you don't have to make more than one trip from the car to your kitchen? That was both of us but on a scooter for an hour-and-a-half-long ride—all that extra weight slowed us down—all the way back to our RV. I have never been flipped off so many times in one day.

You can imagine my excitement when I met a friend who offered to take me on her weekly Whole Foods trips. I had never been to a Whole Foods, and it was tricky to stay on budget, but we did our best. I learned about a lot of new foods, like kombucha, mushroom coffee, and kale chips. I saw terms like *pasture raised* and *grass fed*, which led me to ask questions about why the way an animal is raised might be important. What did it mean for a food to be bioengineered?

New opportunities presented themselves, and Jason and I

changed living arrangements and jobs. With each new place, meeting new people and sharing new experiences, I learned tidbits about healthy eating, like how not all eggs are equal and you should smash your garlic ten minutes before you add it to dishes to maximize its benefits. One of our "opportunities" ended up being rather stressful, and while I did my best to manage my stress, I started experiencing some chronic pain and other symptoms that led me to dive deeper into learning about foods that cause inflammation. I'd thought I was eating whole foods, but I was still consuming too much sugar, low-quality dairy products, refined grains, and seed oils. At this point on the road to becoming crunchy, I was motivated to eat as clean and healthy as I could. But I didn't even think about the chemicals we were confronted with through every other aspect of our lives. Enter: Amy and her knowledge of toxic hand soap.

My journey started before there were influencers as we know them today. In some ways I think it would be easier to start a holistic journey now. There are blogs and people putting themselves in front of a camera to tell you exactly what you're doing wrong and how to make it right.

The problem is, there are *tons* of those people—hundreds of thousands of blogs, Instagram accounts, and YouTube accounts all freely sharing facts, opinions, and opinions posed as fact. There are also legit research studies that are now just a click away. But those research studies can conflict with one another, and depending on the way you phrase your question, the search engine presents different answers. With all this information floating around, different people come to different conclusions, and it's hard to keep up with knowing *all the things*. Not to mention that it feels like the information is constantly changing. Remember back when butter was bad and margarine was king? We also don't know the situations of the people giving the advice. Some seem to have an endless budget, or maybe they're getting paid to push certain "life-changing" products.

The internet has a way of showing off the best in people but bringing out the worst, so sometimes being crunchy can have negative connotations. Health is a delicate topic, and the stance of educating others can come off as judgmental. On the flip side, it's hard to unlearn habits you've had your whole life. Maybe you're already crunchy, maybe you've had an Amy experience, or maybe you are an Amy. I believe that people (crunchy or not) are trying to do the best they can with the information they have. At the root of humanity is a longing for peace, security, and happiness. We are all carrying the baggage of past experiences that have shaped and molded us into who we are. Our memories, stories, and family culture often define why we make the choices we do. People are the way they are for a reason, and it's not right to devalue someone else's experiences because you think you know more or better than they do.

A lot of crunchy people love to research and learn as much as they can, and I think that's where the phrase "Know better, do better" comes from. I cringe when I hear someone use this phrase because it implies that they do, in fact, know better than you, which makes you feel inadequate—and that's an awful feeling. So as you read this book, I hope you don't get a vibe of superiority from me. I am still on this journey of learning. I am not perfect in my choices, and I never will be. What is perfection anyway? Also, I'm well aware that I have been given blessings and opportunities that other people haven't, and I try my best not to take that for granted.

I recently had a conversation with a mom who was questioning the hype around "healthy" food and why crunchy people put restrictions around what they eat. She said, "If it's at the store, it can't be that bad for you. Why would they want to sell you something that's not good for you?" Sadly, some people in powerful positions don't care whether you're making healthy choices; they care about making money. It is up to you to make the decisions that are best for your family. The beautiful thing about life is that we're all different. My best won't necessarily look like your best, and the only person you have to convince that you're doing your best is you. I am not a trained nutritionist, and I don't have a medical degree, but I do have a passion for learning and doing the best I can for my family.

I have come a long way in my crunchy journey, though not as far as Amy, who recently bought a family dairy cow. But I will buy raw milk from her so I can make a homemade version of a Pecan Mudslide.

Remember, your journey won't look the same as anyone else's. Be open to learning some pretty weird things (why yes, there are benefits of drinking the leftover water from your boiled potatoes), but also know your limits and say no to the temptation to compare yourself with anyone else. Ready to explore a crunchy lifestyle? Let's dig in!

What kind of soap do you use in your guest bathroom?

SILKY	SCRUNCHY	REALLY VERY CRUNCHY
Strawberry Pound Cake, with a matching scented candle burning	Something from Trader Joe's made with essential oils	Homemade soap using tallow and breast milk

Jason Says ———————————— ←←←←

Not too many people can say that Root Beer came around to bite them in the butt, but I sure can. In this case, Root Beer was a large spaniel, and I was innocently walking past him to clean a bathroom at a state park when he sank his teeth into my backside. It hurt for days! But not all the results of following Emily's crazy ideas end in scars. All in all, I have to admit this whole crunchy thing has been positive for me and my family. We feel good, probably because we eat right, even if I occasionally grab a burger from my favorite local fast-food joint. But even then, I still order water. From what I've heard, a lot of root beer has corn syrup in it, and apparently that's bad. So I guess if you drink too much of it, root beer could eventually come around to bite you in the butt too.

CHAPTER 3

Anyone Can Be Crunchy

One big misconception is that you have to be within a certain economic demographic to be crunchy. While some variations of being crunchy are expensive, like spending forty-five dollars on three ounces of wild-crafted mushroom tea, there are also plenty of free healthy swaps you can make. For example, you can choose not to put your fruit and vegetables in one of those plastic bags hanging in the produce section. Those things are super frustrating anyway because you can never get them open without licking your fingers. Ditching as much single-use plastic as possible is super crunchy and doesn't cost a dime. To save money, sometimes you have to make sacrifices, like spending more time in the kitchen, because you probably *do* have to be part of a certain financial bracket to justify spending twelve dollars on avocado mayonnaise or ten dollars on organic break-and-bake cookies when you could make those things yourself for a fraction of the price. The biggest sacrifice I've had to make is spending less time consuming entertainment and more time making and doing, but there's an immense satisfaction in seeing what you're able to create, and the money saved is worth the extra work.

Money feels like an icky, taboo topic to discuss. My husband *hates* how much I *love* to talk about money. Neither of us came from money. Both of my parents were raised in poverty. My mom was one of nine children whose sometimes-single mom worked three jobs, so my mom and her siblings were left to raise themselves. My dad, also from a single-parent household, grew up in the projects and ultimately dropped out of high school to enlist in the military in hopes of making a brighter future for himself. My parents had no guidance on money management, and they learned a lot of things the hard way because of it. The truth is, where you come from matters. It matters generally in how your family does things and your perspective on the world and the importance of certain topics, like crunchiness. Financial struggles are often cyclical through generations, and it's hard to focus on "doing better" when you're simply trying to survive.

All that to say, I know what it's like to feel discouraged by financial constraints. There have been so many things I have wanted to do for my family's health that weren't in the budget. For example, I couldn't afford cloth diapers when my first son was born. "But Emily, don't you know cloth diapers will save you money in the long run?" *In the long run.* Those words mean up-front investment, and when you're living paycheck to paycheck, there's no room for investment—even if it means saved money in the long run. Side note: This is one reason I'm such a fan of elimination communication, a method of potty training. It's free (or at least very cheap), but more on that later.

When I first started Really Very Crunchy, I was coming off five years of struggling with feeling inadequate as a "crunchy mom." I followed influencers who seemingly had access to all the latest and greatest supplements, self-care items, and all-in-one cloth diapers. It's easy to take pictures of your aesthetically pleasing home when you have the means to make it that way. I'm not saying those people didn't have to work hard to get where they are (they did), but other people bust their butts day in and day out and don't have financial success to show for it. Having more money makes controlling your environment and your choices easier, but you can still do those things on a budget.

If you're in a season of financial hardship, I hope I can be a beacon of hope and encouragement. Remember, crunchy is a spectrum, and it's all about making the best choices you can where you are—not about being perfect.

One thing that helped me in times of financial strain was to continually remind myself that "comparison is the thief of joy." This is some of the sagest advice I have ever heard. Whether you have it all or you want more, nothing good comes from side-by-side comparisons. You truly cannot know the full extent of someone else's story, especially on the internet, so it's silly to waste your energy comparing yourself to them. Adopt the mentality that you are doing what's best for your nest and they are too. Wouldn't the world be a brighter and more beautiful place if we could all have a generous interpretation of others?

If you're on the side of struggling, embrace where you are and shift your thinking from negative to positive. When my first son was born, I was working as a nanny for a well-off family, and my husband was working as a reporter at a small-town newspaper. I remember thinking, "It's not fair that I can't choose how I dress my child. A baby is a baby only once, and part of the fun of having a baby is getting to pick their clothes!" This woe-is-me mentality will get you nowhere. I decided to shift my perspective to think, "My baby is clothed. My baby is warm. My baby is loved, and my baby doesn't care what he wears. How blessed am I that I can go to a thrift store and find nice clothes for cheap?" Once I changed my perspective, I felt more peace about my financial situation. And, lo and behold, that family gifted me with a huge box of very nice hand-me-downs that their son had outgrown. If you've never experienced it, the joy of getting a big haul of hand-me-downs is up there with college graduation, your wedding day, the birth of your firstborn—we're talking major levels of delight.

Sometimes achieving financial security takes looking at your life and scrutinizing whether you could be allocating money more responsibly to meet your priorities. Are you spending money on subscriptions you don't use? Are you paying a premium for conveniences you could do yourself? How much is your car payment? How much do you spend on getting your hair, nails, and eyelashes done? How much do you spend on alcohol? What about seltzer water? Though, I will admit, drinking seltzer water is a gateway into the crunchy life (one day you're drinking Coke, the next you're sipping

Spindrift, and before you know it, you refuse to drink anything but spring water you bottle yourself directly from the source).

All those things are costly and not necessities. Could you take that money and put it toward buying locally sourced meat or developing a garden or buying natural clothing? Take control of your resources and prioritize what's most important to you.

The Easiest Crunchy Things
You Can Do on the Cheap

- Get outside in the sunshine for fifteen minutes in the morning.
- Add a pinch of salt and a squeeze of lemon to your water.
- Take a walk after meals.
- Bring your own grocery bags to the store.
- Learn to belly breathe.
- Go to bed earlier.
- Choose joy.

There is also the added financial drain of social media consumerism. Before I gained a large social media following, I noticed influencers seemed to be constantly showing off their favorite products. "This glass orb full of crystals is the very best thing I own—I can't imagine my life without it. You, too, need this orb so you can feel all the amazing benefits. My existence was sad before I owned this orb." I was intrigued by a product that claimed to improve your entire life, including sleep. Especially when so many influencers professed it was the best thing ever. It cost $1,000, so it was definitely out of our budget, even for crystal-filled orbs, but that didn't mean I didn't want it. Sure enough, once my channel reached fifty thousand followers, the orb company reached out to me wanting to send me my very own orb. A $1,000 product for free! I could even try it out for sixty days before posting anything to my platform because they were certain the life-changing benefits would be so noticeable that I'd want to tell everyone about it, plus I could make a decent commission for every orb sold through my link.

Maybe I didn't have it plugged in right, but the glass orb did nothing to change my life. Coming from a history of not being able to afford pricey items, I found it kind of hard to send back something so luxurious. But I learned very quickly that influencers get cool, expensive stuff for free. Some of the stuff might be legitimately great! But as a consumer, be careful about who you follow and the message they are sending. If anyone tells you your health and happiness hinge on obtaining a certain product, be wary. I have no idea what other influencers purchase or what they are given, but from this side of things, I've become a lot more cautious about believing something is a must-have.

At the end of the day, you could be the richest person in the world and still not be crunchy enough for some people. That's why it's important to do what's best for you and your family and make decisions in the micro rather than in the macro. Little decisions over time make a big difference. Maybe today you decide to eat fruit instead of chips. Maybe you devote more time to being outside instead of in front of a screen. A lot of crunchy decisions cost very little—or absolutely nothing.

You have to eat at a gas station and have only five dollars. What do you buy?

SILKY	SCRUNCHY	REALLY VERY CRUNCHY
Cool Ranch Doritos and a big blue slushy	A beef stick and a can of LaCroix	In-season fruit and a glass bottle of mountain spring water

Jason Says ─────────────── -«««-

I'm gonna shoot it to you straight. Sometimes being crunchy can save you money. Yeah, you might have to spring for the pasture-raised chicken or the raw milk that one guy sells out of the back of his van, but I can tell you this: the crunchy mom isn't asking for diamonds on any special occasion. If you ever see Emily with a diamond ring on, well, I found that diamond in the dirt when I was a kid and saved it until I married her. You tell me a crunchier way to get someone a diamond. I'll wait. Also, think about how often some women get their hair and nails done. Do you know how much that costs? There are enough artificial fragrances in those places to give a crunchy mom a headache for a month. The thing is, though, when it is time to get her a gift or do something nice for her, you've got to reach deep and truly think about what makes her happy. Bonus points if you thrifted that special gift for next to nothing. In these cases, it truly is the thought that counts.

SECTION 2

The Crunchy Basics

CHAPTER 4

The Basic Needs (Part 1)

I can't believe Mrs. Quartermouse had any influence on my crunchy journey, as she was the type of old lady whose hair had a blue hue from some sort of chemical concoction she called a "rinse." You knew right when you walked into school that Mrs. Quartermouse was subbing because everywhere she went, she left a scent that could be described as one part mothballs, one part mung beans, and two parts Chanel no. 5. She wore blue eyeshadow to match her hair and passed out "quarter bucks" for good behavior, claiming you could use them to get out of homework or detention or as bonus points, but none of the teachers accepted them as a usable form of currency. Nonetheless, she did teach me that when you don't know what to do, you should KISS: keep it simple, stupid. I always felt slightly offended by that last *stupid* thrown in there, but that's just my inner everyone-gets-a-trophy millennial talking.

Society has done everything in its power to complicate our lives. Busyness is a status symbol likened to wealth. Wealth is more important than ever because you have to look your best—be your best—all the time. There's a product, pill, or procedure to fix any problem you might encounter. We want more out of our lives, and we want it now because we deserve it! Mr. Rogers, that dear old man, once said, "Our society is much more interested in information than wonder, in noise rather than silence."[1] I believe the Grinch highlights this best when he says, "Oh, the Noise! Noise! Noise! Noise!"[2] Am I allowed to fuse quotes from Mr. Rogers and the Grinch like that? What I'm trying to say is, the journey to living a more holistic, crunchy life is often a journey to simplicity.

As with any lifestyle, there are people who will try to sell you things and claim you need this or that if you want to be healthy. In reality, it's best to break the crunchy lifestyle down to KIS (I'll leave out the *stupid* for you because that's what friends do): What are the basic needs for survival, and how can you make the best choices to meet those needs? It was in my middle school social studies class, with Mrs. Quartermouse subbing, that I learned about Maslow's hierarchy of needs. You've likely seen this visual before: a pyramid with physiological needs at the bottom, then safety and security, moving up to love and belonging, then to self-esteem, all topped by self-actualization. Physiological needs are the ones for basic survival, a good place to start if you're looking to make changes toward living a more holistic life. This pyramid is not to be confused with the food pyramid that we were taught growing up, which was terribly flawed and messed up a lot of people's views on food, but we can touch on that later.

Your physiological needs include but are not limited to the following: air, water, food, clothing, shelter, and sleep. How can you make changes in each of these areas to remove toxins that may negatively impact your health and wellness? We'll discuss some options throughout the remainder of this chapter and the next.

First, I want to acknowledge that having access to these things is an incredible blessing and a privilege that is not lost on me. I have had struggles in my life, but not once have I worried where my next meal would come from. Even when my husband and I were below the poverty level, we always had food available. I want to be sensitive to all walks of life, so before we dive into the ways you can make your physiological needs crunchier, let me say this: you know your limits, and no one else can define them for you. Crunchiness is a spectrum, and it won't look the same for everyone—there is no single best way. Do what's best for you.

1. Air

Is air really just air? Dioxins, benzene, vinyl chloride, cadmium, and lead make up some of the 188 hazardous air pollutants that can be found in our air.[3] From coughing to cancer to congenital disabilities, polluted air can have myriad adverse effects on our health.[4]

Would this even be a crunchy book if I didn't include a quote by John Muir, Ralph Waldo Emerson, or Henry David Thoreau? For the purposes of this chapter, I'm going with Emerson's "Live in the sunshine, swim the sea / Drink the wild air's salubrity,"[5] but I cannot guarantee the nature-driven, thought-provoking quotes will end here. You can blame the 1990s for me living my life through the lens of an epic motivational poster.

According to the EPA, "Air within homes and other buildings can be more seriously polluted than the outdoor air in even the largest and most industrialized cities. . . . The risks to health may be greater due to exposure to air pollution indoors than outdoors." On average, Americans spend 90 percent of their time indoors.[6] How many of those 188 hazardous pollutants are in your home? It is nearly impossible to test for every toxin, but I do know that if you want to breathe cleaner air, you need to get outside. Listen to Emerson and drink the wild air! I'll never forget the January day a newspaper reporter sheepishly approached my son and me as we played on the playground of a local park. "Mind if I take your picture for the paper?" My husband had previously been a reporter, so I knew this meant it must have been a slow news cycle, but it still tickled me that a toddler playing outside in the cold was newsworthy. To make it even funnier, his picture made the front page!

I know being outside may not always be practical (unless you're Scandinavian and have it all figured out), but there are a few things you can do to clear the air inside. The cheapest and easiest option is to open the windows. Opening your windows allows indoor pollutants to escape. Obviously, there are caveats, like if you live in a highly polluted area with lots of traffic or near a factory, in which case you should open your windows for just fifteen minutes during a low-traffic time. But letting in fresh air can only do so much. Sometimes you have to make changes from within.

Were you ever broken up with in high school? You knew what was about to happen. You saw the warning signs. You stood face-to-face, the awkwardness so thick in the air that it became hard to breathe. Your heart started racing. Heaven forbid you were wearing an antiperspirant (aluminums!), but if you were, it kicked in (hopefully). You tried to brace yourself as you waited for the harsh truth: the two of you weren't meant to be.

This may very well be the hardest part of your crunchy journey, but it's time for a breakup. It's time for you to break up with fragrances.

Fragrances are everywhere. Why do we need our trash cans to smell like "fresh linen"? Is it really necessary for your toilet paper to smell like chamomile? An average person is confronted with hundreds of fragrances every day. The word *fragrance* on a product covers dozens, sometimes hundreds, of chemicals that make up that fragrance. That little word is on shampoo, lotion, soap, makeup, serums, deodorant, dish soap, laundry detergent, dryer sheets, cleaners—to name a few. And then there are the items with the sole purpose of adding more fragrance into the world: perfume, room sprays, air fresheners, candles. Scented goods drastically add to indoor air pollution. We are talking about thousands of chemicals, some of which contain phthalates, some of which are endocrine disruptors, which can cause reproductive and developmental toxicity, respiratory issues such as asthma, or even cancer. Yes, some fragrances contain carcinogens, which are compounds known to cause cancer, and companies don't have to disclose which toxic concoction they are using as long as they add the word *fragrance* to a list of ingredients. All these risks because we like the smell.

"Cashmere Woods" are not a real thing; woods smell like dirt and moss. Hawaii doesn't smell like the marketed "Hawaiian Breeze"; it probably smells like sweaty tourists. And "Crisp Waters," in reality, smell a little bit like fish. I know, I know, it's a harsh reality. Once you're done sobbing, come back to me, and I'll help you feel a little better.

First, you need to know you have been lied to. Cleanliness is not determined by the smell of something. Fragrances don't improve a product's performance. Trash bags that have no scent are just as good at holding trash (just get a trash can with a lid and you won't even notice), and dish soap that is fragrance-free is still able to wash your dishes. Your home can still be clean even if it doesn't smell like fresh lemon zest or a pine forest. If you do only one thing to step into the crunchy-verse, I'd implore you to give up fragrances.

This can seem daunting if everything in your house contains fragrances. I'm not a health expert; I'm a mom on a mission to provide the healthiest home for my family, and what I'm about to say may be odd to the hard-core crunchies out there. But here it is: if you don't have the means to throw away everything and start fresh, don't. Everything (crunchy or not) is so expensive, and it's not worth putting a financial strain on your family. That is, unless you're experiencing respiratory symptoms; then maybe go ahead and ditch all the fragranced things. However, if you're looking to make switches for long-term health impacts, the next time you go to buy something, look for the most natural version of that product. You can always check out the reels of your favorite Instagram influencers if you need an idea for a product swap. I'll list some of my favorite social media accounts and other resources in the resources section of this book.

If you can't bear the thought of life without smells, consider swapping to the natural version of your favorite smells. Love the smell of lavender? Hang up bundles of dried lavender or even make sachets and stick them around your house. Put fresh herbs next to your door so they're the first thing you smell when you walk in. Burn beeswax candles for a warm-honey smell. The scent of pine needles simmering in a pot of water on the stove beats the smell of Pine-Sol any day. You don't have to live scent-free to live added fragrance–free.

If you do make the fragrance switch, and especially if you do it all at once, be aware that it may be difficult for you to smell the natural scents. Scented candles, toilet sprays, dish soaps—all of them are more intense than the natural versions they claim to emulate. So at first you may not notice your beeswax candles are giving off a smell. But give it time. The longer you are away from artificial fragrances, the more your sense of smell will acclimate to the versions nature has provided. In the reverse, and especially in my experience, artificial scents become way too harsh on the nose. If I get too much of a whiff, an artificial scent can give me a headache. For some reason this has been especially true with laundry detergents and perfumes. We have all come across the old lady who forgot how many pumps of perfume she sprayed, so she pumped just a few more. Imagine walking into that cloud after you've given up all fragrances. That sensitivity may seem like a downside at first, but then you think about having that fake scent all around you or even on you all the time—wearing it, sleeping in it, constantly breathing in these thousands of lab-created chemicals meant to fake a smell found in nature—and the trade-off doesn't seem so bad.

I've also had great success by typing into a search engine "nontoxic swap for _____." There are countless trusted, reliable sources that can help educate you about the products you're using and how they might impact your air quality and your health. The best way to educate yourself is to start reading and questioning labels. Companies are allowed to sell phthalates and carcinogens, so it's up to you to wade through the noise. In the fashion of capitalizing on opportunities, companies can make their products look healthier in an effort to trick people who want to switch to more natural products. This is called greenwashing. Just because something says "plant based," "made with essential oils," or "all natural" doesn't make it healthy. One tiny healthy or green part of their product does not outweigh all the harmful aspects. Greenwashing is misleading and unethical, and if a company is intentionally misrepresenting their product, it's probably not a good product to be using.

You don't have to invest in fancy cleaning systems. You can keep your home clean using vinegar, baking soda, and Bon Ami. That's all you need, and you can buy all three for under five dollars each. Think about how your great-grandmother cared for her home. You don't need a bunch of ritzy-glitzy stuff to get the job done. Remember KIS: simplicity is often the crunchiest option available.

Aside from ditching fragrances and opening your windows, other ways to keep your air clean include vacuuming regularly, minimizing indoor pets (please don't hate me), running an air purifier, and having your air ducts cleaned. The size of your home, its age and architectural style, and the materials used to build your house also influence air quality as well as the home's overall crunch factor.

One of the biggest things to be aware of in your home's makeup is mold. Whatever you do, try to avoid living in a home that has mold. Mold can cause a ton of awful health issues, including allergies and asthma. Some things to look out for are visible mold spores, a musty or damp smell, and areas of water damage like squishy floors or wavy walls. If you're having what seems like a seasonal allergy that never seems to go away, that could be a sign of mold. If you suspect a mold problem in your house, the best thing to do is have it inspected by a professional, as they know what to look for and where to look. They can also tell you if it is spreading and the best ways to try to prevent it, which almost always includes keeping moisture-prone areas of your home dry since mold thrives with moisture.

Mold isn't only lurking behind walls. Sometimes we don't even know we're being exposed to mold or harmful mycotoxins (a mold by-product). Sometimes it's hiding in our food. Raisins and other dried fruits, grape juice, peanut butter, and even coffee are often riddled with mycotoxins.

As a crunchy momma, I want to use as many natural products in my home as possible. Sometimes I'm tempted to take the quick and easy route, but the crunchy way generally isn't the easiest or most convenient. I was especially tempted when we bought our current home. Our house was a for-sale-by-owner, very outdated diamond in the rough that was built in 1981. The kitchen had parquet wood carpet—yes, carpet made to look like wood . . . in the kitchen. We have slowly made updates when we've been able to afford them. A piece of trim is still missing above the refrigerator from our DIY kitchen renovation a couple of years ago. Our bathroom still features a pea soup–green sink with a coordinating shower. The first thing I did when we moved in was replace the pea soup–green toilet because I can live with a lot, but I draw the line there.

Along with the faux parquet floors, our kitchen had to be gutted because, and I can't believe I'm telling you this, it was infested with roaches. Every time we viewed our home before buying, the seller insisted on being there. This should have been a tip-off that something wasn't right, but we figured since it was for sale by owner, he hung around to unlock and lock the place. In reality, he must have gone in and banged all the cabinets to warn the roaches of our coming before we did our inspection. When we moved in, we cleaned everything thoroughly and didn't notice traces of pests, but it was dark in there and hard to tell if the cabinets were just a little crusty.

A couple of days into living there, I opened our silverware drawer to see *hundreds* of freshly hatched baby roaches crawling all over our utensils. Screaming ensued. We started grabbing all the drawers and carrying them outside. I distinctly remember shouting at Jason, "Call Terminix! Tell them to bomb the place! *Wait, no—tell them to burn it to the ground!*" Thankfully, my parents live in the same city as we do (we chose to move back here so we could have a support system when we had kids), so we were able to squish into their guest bedroom while kitchen renovations took place at our house. I was seriously debating whether to use a pest control company until I read a study in an American Academy of Pediatrics publication that concluded that childhood exposure to indoor insecticides was linked to a nearly 50 percent increased risk of childhood leukemia and lymphoma.[7] I decided I'd rather take my chances with roach-carried illnesses, but thankfully, there's almost always a way to take care of a problem without using dangerous chemicals. Does PETA advocate for roaches? If so, they may not like the advice I'm going to give now: boric acid. The natural-alternative answer for roaches is boric acid. It worked like a charm (read about it and use caution). We haven't seen a single sign of roaches in the three years since. PS: If your three-year-old knows there are roaches in your kitchen, so will everyone you meet.

I know as well as anyone that you don't have control over *all the things.* Jason and I have found ourselves in some unique positions over the years of crunch-ifying our lives, and when I say "unique," I don't mean "glamorous." We have learned that having an artesian well sounds fancy but means your water might smell like rotten eggs. We have learned that you can get rid of mice using massive amounts of dried tansy, bay leaves, peppermint, and lots and lots of prayer. We have learned that just because a flea-infested dog moves out of a place doesn't mean the fleas go with it. Most importantly, we have learned that sometimes you have to make the best of where you are, roach infestation and all.

2. Water

When we were full-time RVers, our vehicle decided to overheat while traveling through the Mojave Desert in July. I grew up with old vehicles, and I remembered my dad telling me to blast the heat in the cab to help cool an overheating engine. I don't know if that was good advice, but it's what we chose to do. So there we were, blasting the heat, in July, in the desert, when we decided we needed to pull over to see if we could get the RV to cool down naturally. We felt stranded. There was nothing around. No cell signal. We didn't even have smartphones at this point in our lives, and we were using a shoestring and a road atlas to map our trips. Our poor dog, a collie with the thickest, hottest coat imaginable, started looking uncomfortable as we sat there low-key panicking. So I opened her water container that we always had ready when traveling. As she lapped up the sweet, cool H_2O, I, too, started to feel thirsty. I went to the fridge with high hopes even though I knew the truth: there was nothing in our fridge. We chose not to pack anything to eat or drink because we'd planned to stop by a grocery store somewhere along the way. But there had been nothing along the way.

My thirst magnified at this realization. I would've drunk

from the dog bowl if I hadn't loved my dog too much to take her refreshment. My really very crunchy persona maybe even would have allowed me to try to drink from the lead-free hose if I could shake some water from it. Never the lead-laden one though. My brother lived in Joshua Tree at the time, and that was where we were heading, so we decided to push the engine (with the heat blasting) until we got to his place. Once we arrived, we were able to get the RV to a repair shop, where the mechanic informed us that our temperature gauge was broken and our engine was perfectly fine. Wasn't it Leonardo da Vinci who said, "Water is the driving force of all nature"? It certainly was our force to drive on a fake hot engine. I will never take water for granted after that close call with thirsting to death.

We all need water, but is water simply water anymore? A nine-month investigation by the *Guardian* and Consumer Reports showed evidence that it's not as pure as one would hope. More than 35 percent of the samples tested showed high level of PFAS, which are forever chemicals.[8] Forever chemicals are exactly what they sound like, chemicals that don't break down in our bodies or our environment. They are forever, and we all know forever is a very long time. These chemicals are everywhere—clothes (I'm looking at you, yoga pants), bedding, backpacks, tents, car seats, and furniture all commonly contain PFAS. PFAS are linked to learning delays in children, various types of cancer, and immunosuppression. If we are confronted with PFAS in every other area of our lives, why would we also want to be drinking them? This investigation also found arsenic in some water, and a total of 118 out of 120 samples tested showed levels of lead.[9] Exposure to arsenic increases your chances of cancer. Lead exposure is unsafe at any level and is linked to brain and nervous system dysfunction.

Aside from that study, here's a list of other hazardous things commonly found in tap water:

- Heavy metals,[10] including chromium, cadmium, mercury, copper, and aluminum (it's pretty bad when all those things make up one bullet point instead of being separated out)
- Microplastics[11]
- PFAS (those pesky forever chemicals)
- Herbicides and pesticides (yes, those have *s*'s on the end of them)
- Bacteria, viruses, and parasites
- Chlorine treatment byproducts
- Arsenic
- Nitrates
- Radioactive contaminants
- Vinyl Chloride
- Perchlorate
- Pharmaceuticals[12]

One hot-topic debate I didn't mention on that list is fluoride. Fluoride is known to be effective in preventing tooth decay. It is also a known neurotoxin and can have a variety of health consequences when consumed at certain levels. Are those levels high enough in the community drinking water to be a concern? There are laws in place regulating the amount of fluoride that can be added. Personally, I don't want to risk consuming it, but the main reason I am anti fluorinated water is that added fluoride does nothing for the quality of water. Adding fluoride takes away some freedom of choice because fluoride is added to water as a form of mass "medication" to treat the general public's teeth. If someone wants to use fluoride, they can do so with toothpaste (though there are natural options for tooth remineralization such as hydroxyapatite).

The idea of mass medication sounds more menacing than I mean. Am I saying I believe the government is using fluoride in water sources to control your mind? I'll leave that one for the conspiracy theorists. But do I like the idea of my health being influenced for the sake of the general population's dental health? Also no. You don't have to be an extremist to have an opinion.

On the Topic of Dental Health

Floss is a major source of PFAS and plastic waste.[13] There are tons of natural flosses out there, ranging from silk to bamboo. You can also practice tongue scraping for fighting bad breath.

What do you think of when I say charcoal? Please don't say those toxic briquettes for grilling. Your answer should be "charcoal powder," and you can use it for whitening your teeth instead of those plastic whitening strips.

The good news is, water free from all the hazardous additives is accessible to almost everyone. You don't have to have a whole home filter for your water—you can buy a pitcher or even a countertop filter that will take out a lot of yucky stuff.

3. Food

We all know the saying "You are what you eat," and I'm tempted to invoke that here, but the crunchy way of eating is high in quality fats, pasture-raised meats, and ferments, so to say that would be to say you should eat to become a fat wild animal who smells rotten. That's no way to convince someone to consider a lifestyle switch.

As a side note, sauerkraut and kimchi smell rotten, but that doesn't mean they taste rotten. No one gives cheese connoisseurs a hard time for liking things that stink. I do have some advice from a non–cheese connoisseur: don't try blue cheese for the first time on a cruise ship. I'm speaking from personal experience, and I'm not sure I can ever fully enjoy blue cheese as it is forever tinged with the memory of the first impression I received upon the *Wonder of the Seas*. The flavor of rotten blue cheese is biting.

Other Lessons I Learned on That Cruise

1. Don't go swimming when you're in a storm and the boat is causing the swimming pool to shift so

much you can see the ground where the deep end
is supposed to be. It was dangerously fun though.
2. Older people are more fun to hang out with than
young people.
3. The midnight pizza buffet is never a good idea.

Food is a huge part of our lives. We all need to eat to survive. As with every topic of wellness, it can get a little tricky when you start choosing to go against the average, acceptable norm for the sake of wanting to *do better*. I cringe as I type those words because *doing better* insinuates life is a competition and you are trying to do better than those around you, but what I mean by that is do better for yourself. Make better choices for you and your family, no matter what stage of life you're in. As with anything, you can take the focus of healthy eating too far where you become afraid of certain foods. This is called orthorexia. Do not be afraid of food. It's good to make healthy choices, but if making healthy choices (or an occasional not-so-healthy choice) causes mental distress, you may want to seek professional help. I try to be intentional about not making any foods an enemy, but rather being aware of and understanding the nourishment and benefits, or lack thereof, in foods I consume.

A lot of talk about food can get muddled with words and phrases that are a bit confusing, but fear not. Here are a few words and phrases you can throw out in conversation to ensure that you sound like you know what you're talking about:

Inflammation: The kryptonite of the crunchy person, inflammation is the biological response against harmful stimuli such as toxins, bacteria, and food dyes.

Immune response: The crunchy obsession with having a good immune system goes hand in hand with having as little inflammation as possible. Bonus words in this category include elderberry syrup, fire cider, and fermented honey and garlic.

Microbiome: The trophy of a crunchy person, the microbiome should be rich and diverse. It is the bacteria that naturally live in and on our bodies and play a mega role in our health.

Lacto-fermentation: This is an easy form of fermenting vegetables that, when consumed, increase the diversity of the ever-important gut microbiome.

Natural and artificial flavorings: Crunchy people want their food to taste how it tastes without having to alter the flavor, so none of these please. I know it's tricky because *natural* sounds natural. Really, it means part of the flavor was extracted from a natural source, but the result of the "natural flavoring" was still manipulated in a lab and often contains synthetic chemicals, preservatives, solvents, and emulsifiers added during the production process. How else do you think they get beaver anus to taste like raspberries? Just saying.

Seed oils: These are the bane of the crunchy person's existence. Seed oils (including safflower, corn, soybean, canola, and cottonseed) all contribute to inflammation (refer back to the first point in this list).

Nose to tail: This means eating animal fats and organs. This is how our ancestors used to eat, not wasting any part of animals for food. Organ meats are full of nutrients, vitamins, and minerals that are easily digested and processed by our bodies.

Bioavailability: A food may have a lot of nutrients and minerals, but our bodies aren't able to access all the nutrients in digestion. Bioavailable food allows our bodies to access its many health benefits. Still sounds a little pompous at times, even if it's true.

If you've been around the health food world at all, you'll see that people refer to healthy eating as a lifestyle instead of a diet. A diet connotes something restrictive and is usually based on a timed goal. A lifestyle change is something deeper and more sustainable. The goal of healthy eating isn't to deprive yourself of all the things you love, but rather to shift your relationship with food and enlighten yourself on truly nourishing your body rather than merely feeding it.

The grocery store is where you make many important decisions for your family. Processed foods have been linked to obesity, type 2 diabetes,[14] heart disease,[15] irritable bowel syndrome,[16] and an increased risk of cancer.[17] Processed foods don't just affect your physical health, they are also linked to dementia, depression, anxiety, and other mood disorders.[18] In my opinion, the ease and convenience of these foods aren't worth the risks and the degradation of your health. You only get one body—treat it well by feeding it well.

One of the most important things you can do for your

health is to eat mostly whole foods. This means you should try to choose as many foods as you can that can be recognized as something naturally occurring. I've heard it said that you shouldn't eat anything that your great-grandmother wouldn't recognize as food (that is, highly processed, prepackaged items that have ingredient lists longer than my arm). Foods that have to be fortified with vitamins and nutrients aren't naturally healthy for you. Buy foods that provide vitamins and nutrients without the need for fortification. When you do buy packaged foods, look for items made up of ingredients you could find in a pantry, ones with whole-food ingredients. If you look at the ingredients and don't know what something is, you probably shouldn't be eating it.

The easiest way to choose healthy foods is to stick to the outside aisles of the grocery store. Fresh produce, meat, and dairy are all on the outskirts of the store. If you keep yourself from going up and down aisles, you remove the temptation to buy overly processed foods. If you are into taking baby steps, the way my husband and I started minimizing our consumption of processed foods was to buy packaged items only when they contained five ingredients or less. Minimizing your intake of processed foods is a fantastic way to improve your health and hopefully longevity. Sometimes this takes planning; cooking in bulk and freezing the extra meals to make when you don't have time to cook is super helpful.

Do the best you can with the resources you have. I'm not a nutritionist, so all I can do is speak from personal experience. It's up to you to dig in and discover what foods are best for you. There are lots of different diets and lifestyles that may benefit different body types. There is no one-size-fits-all diet, but a few you might want to check out include the Weston A. Price Dietary Guidelines, paleo, and Whole30. All of these focus on whole, nutrient-dense foods.

There's a lot of debate on whether you should eat organic food. Some people say it's a scam and not worth the money; others claim it's extremely important for food quality. There is limited research on the matter. The conspiracy crunchy mom within me says, "Follow the money, honey. Big Ag, Big Pharma, and Big Dairy all want your cash, so why would they support research that exposes their way of doing things? But there are loopholes with organic farms, and some of them aren't entirely honest, so it really is all about money. Big Organic is a thing now too. Trust no one." Conspiracy Crunchy Mom complicates everything, but then I remember: KIS. Seek out simplicity when you don't know the answer. In my nonconspiratorial opinion, the best you can do is seek out farms in your area and talk to them about their growing practices. With the rising interest in growing and raising nutritional foods, you may even be able to find a regenerative farm: the gold standard of farming these days.

Food is expensive, and I know it can be discouraging when you can't afford to buy the quality of food you want. When I couldn't afford local, pasture-raised eggs, I knew any egg was better for me than buying canned biscuits. The further your food is from its natural state, the less healthy it is for you. Organic or not, the key is to invest your dollars into whole, nutrient-dense foods. These foods are not only better for you but also more satiating than boxed and processed foods. If you must have snacks, consider making them yourself. If you can buy it at the store, you can likely make it at home—except Cheetos. I'm pretty sure no home chef can rival the chemical concoction of those crispy-yet-fluffy, crunchy bites of goodness. They make a greenwashed version: Cheetos Simply Puffs. They're not great for you, but I'll admit to buying a bag (or two) so I could experience the delight of licking cheese powder off my fingers. Don't tell anyone, though; I have a reputation to maintain.

Homemade Snack Ideas

The following list includes easy things you can make (with just a few ingredients) to up your crunch. Check the ingredient labels on these foods and you'll see how many unnecessary things are in the store-bought versions.

- **Crackers**—All it takes is flour, water, olive oil, and salt
- **Yogurt**—Milk and a little yogurt starter, and you're set
- **Bread**—Flour, water, yeast, and salt
- **Bone broth**—Bones, water, and a splash of apple cider vinegar
- **Salad dressings**—Oil and vinegar with other add-ins, like mustard
- **Mayonnaise**—Eggs, oil, and salt
- **Granola** (Can I even be crunchy without suggesting this one?)—Oats, coconut oil, maple syrup, and add-ins like nuts or dried fruit

There are ways to get the gold standard of food without having to fork over gold for it. When we lived in Wisconsin, I volunteered as a worker at Springdale Farm, a beautiful organic farm run by the kindest people. In exchange for my help packing boxes, I got a community-supported agriculture (CSA) subscription of freshly grown, organic produce. And there were often extras of certain things you could load up on. I have never met a farmer who couldn't use more hands, so although it takes a little courage to call and ask, don't be afraid to see if you can exchange work for products. You can check wwoofusa.org (wwoof.net for the rest of the world) to find an organic farm that you can contact. Another farming opportunity was when I spent a whole day shoveling trenches in the mud and helped my friend, owner of Tulip Lane, plant thirty thousand tulips in exchange for a subscription to her seasonal flower CSA. I not only got the satisfaction of enjoying cut flowers all spring but also got to go out to the patch and see a huge field of beautiful flowers that I helped plant. Be bold and ask. The worst someone can do is say no.

And sometimes you will be rejected. An old bachelor who lives on my block owns about an acre of woods next to his home. We are familiar with most of our neighbors because we take a walk around the neighborhood every evening after dinner. This man has been friendly enough to wave back when my kids say hello and smile when they ride their bikes by his house. One day while he was out chopping wood, I mentioned that I noticed the border of his acre of woods was covered with blackberry bushes. He said yes, they were delicious, but there was no way he could eat all of them. I took that as an opportunity to ask if the boys and I could come pick some once they were ripe. He just stared at me, but I knew he had heard what I asked. He turned around and went right back to chopping wood. Thinking maybe he felt uncomfortable telling me no, I said some version of "Okay, bye!" The next day he was bush hogging all the blackberry bushes. It was awkward to say the least, but it won't stop me from asking others in the future!

I won't pretend like the only thing we eat as a treat is foraged blackberries from somewhere other than my neighbor's yard. We aren't perfect in any sense of the word, and sometimes nostalgia gets the better of us. When Jason and I were in college and dating, we used to love the television show *Lost*. Once per week we would head to Culver's, then meet all our friends at my apartment to watch the latest episode together. There's something so delightfully sentimental about going there and getting a vanilla custard to share, even if it does have corn syrup in it. So, on very special occasions, we will go grab one together. (*Insert sweating emoji here.*) I remember being so embarrassed after I started making videos about being crunchy because one of the employees recognized me and asked to have her picture taken with me. My cover was blown. I just knew she'd post that picture of me and all my followers would know I wasn't perfectly crunchy all the time. My loving husband had to remind me that perfection isn't the goal. I like to ask myself: What is the general rule of our family? If the general rule is that we cook nourishing meals at home, it's okay to occasionally make an exception to the rule.

My first video to go viral was about "my worst nightmare" of getting invited to a kid's birthday party. I'll be honest, it sort of does feel nightmarish anytime we're invited to such events; I don't want to be a controlling mom who "deprives" her children of all the junk food when other kids get to partake so freely. But I also don't want to encourage my kids to consume the very foods I work to keep out of our home. I found myself dwelling on my kids' food choices at parties, and I don't want them to pick up on that because I think anxiety is far more damaging than a little bit of soybean oil and food dye (unless there's a true allergy, obviously).

So I decided to give my kids a choice when we attend those types of events. A day or so ahead of time, I say, "Hey, so-and-so's birthday party is coming up. You are totally welcome to partake in party treats, but I want you to know that we can make alternatives if you'd like." My older son is pretty in tune with his body for a six-year-old and knows, from experience, junk food doesn't make him feel great, so every time I have offered an alternative, he has taken it. Honestly, what kid doesn't want to choose his own favorite treat anyway? And every time we have done this, the only response he has gotten from other kids is that they want what he's having. Thanks to the rise in food allergies, there are tons of allergen-friendly (that is, typically a little bit "cleaner") fun options out there. There are sprinkles colored with spirulina and beet juice and natural options for food dye. Trying to choose healthier options doesn't mean you can't have fun.

Ways to Throw a Really Very Crunchy
Birthday Party

- Use party decorations that can be used again and again. We have a birthday banner made out of upcycled wool sweaters that we pull out for each birthday party. Start collecting tablecloths that can be washed instead of single-use plastic ones. Say no to balloons.
- Make the cake from scratch instead of buying store-bought cakes or cupcakes. Use natural dyes and sprinkles to make it extra fun. Serve one sweet treat; the rest of the food can be fruits, vegetables, and healthy alternatives.
- Serve water and freshly squeezed lemonade instead of sodas.
- If possible, use plates and cups from your home instead of disposables.
- Encourage kids to bring secondhand toys, games, and books instead of buying new ones.
- Ditch the goody bags and make a craft together for kids to take home instead.

4. Clothing

You're probably thinking, "Fragrances, indoor insecticides, poison in the tap water, seed oils in everything else. What's next? Are you going to strip the very clothes off my back? And my answer is: I might.

I'm kidding. Sort of. It would really depend on what you're wearing.

Clothing is a basic need. People wear clothes all the time, aside from the 80 percent of guys who mow their lawns shirtless. But let's assume most people wear clothes most of the time. One of the biggest negative impacts we are making on our planet and our health comes from the idea that we need to have clothes aligned with the latest and greatest fashion trend. A dozen or more documentaries highlight the atrocities of fast fashion: how it is bad for our environment and our health. Like anything else you put on your body, clothes can impact your health. Study after study shows that polyester underwear is detrimental to sperm count in men.[19] Aside from the concern of shedding microplastics that we breathe, clothes are sprayed with and made up of toxic chemicals including formaldehydes, pesticides, azo dyes, PFAS, flame retardants, and even heavy metals such as lead.

Your skin is your largest organ, and what's rubbing it all day long affects your health. At the time of writing this book, there was a recall on Disney-themed clothing from a brand called Bentex because of a risk of lead poisoning. This brand is carried at places like Amazon and T.J. Maxx. Who doesn't love shopping at T.J. Maxx? There you are, thinking you picked up a cute little Minnie Mouse outfit for your little mini me to wear to a playdate, and then, *bam*, you find out you paid $12.99 for the risk of lead poisoning.[20] Sometimes I wish I lived in the caveman days because at least back then you knew what was dangerous. Sure, you had to worry about saber-toothed cats, wolves, and giant man-eating birds, but lead-laced Elsa shirts just weren't the same issue they are today. Oh, and toxic mushrooms. As an avid forager, I'm so thankful for those who figured out which mushrooms were deadly so I didn't have to. When you consider the hidden poison both in our princess tees and on our forest floors, assessing danger would have been *way* easier back in the prehistoric period.

Is anything safe? Yes. In pretty much every choice you make, there is a more natural version of the product. Cotton, linen, silk, wool, and hemp are fibers produced from plants or animals. I prefer to choose fibers that don't require a lot of pesticides to grow: wool, linen, and hemp. Sometimes these fibers are more expensive when you're buying them new, but often they are also more durable. I like to try to buy fewer but more timeless pieces that I can wear for a long time. A friend of mine in her eighties told me that every spring when she was a kid, her parents gave her a new dress for Easter Sunday. That was her church dress for the year. For the year! Think about all the Sunday morning arguments, all the stress of trying to make it to church on time, that could be avoided if we all had our one Sunday outfit. That might be too extreme for you, but maybe you could think about choosing natural materials that are more durable and healthier for you and your family.

Fabrics You Should Avoid

- **Polyester**—Made of plastic and treated with tons of toxic chemicals, including forever chemicals, that rub off on your skin
- **Acrylic**—Made of plastic, known to shed microplastics easily
- **Rayon**—Treated with toxic chemicals and, like all synthetic materials, very bad for the environment to produce
- **Acetate**—Requires extensive chemical processing
- **Nylon**—Petroleum-based fiber that receives a laundry list of chemical treatments

Unless you're a toddler, I'm sure you know by now the world doesn't revolve around you, but the choices you make can impact our world. Okay, maybe not the choices you alone make, but if we all decided to make more sustainable choices, we could make a difference together. Saying no to fast fashion isn't just about your health—it's about our environment. Fast fashion contributes to water pollution, soil pollution, and rain forest degradation in the areas where clothes are manufactured. The fashion industry is also well known for violating human rights by providing poor working conditions and using child labor. It's our responsibility to make ethical choices whenever possible. People own more clothes today than they ever have, and those clothes are ending up in the dump within a year of purchasing.[21] Think about all the wasted energy in the production of clothes: from transporting them from the other side of the world all the way down to the heating and cooling of the massive stores where they sit waiting to be purchased. Almost all of it just for the clothes to be thrown in the garbage. Trash aside, a recent study suggests that 85 percent of man-made pollution on ocean shorelines is the result of microfiber shedding from the fast-fashion industry's synthetic textiles.[22]

An Incomplete List of Stores That Sell
Fast Fashion

- Zara
- H&M
- Forever 21
- ASOS
- SHEIN
- UNIQLO[23]
- You get the drift.

I suppose I don't envy cavemen. I mean, I got to grow up in a quintessential 1990s household. A time when sugary cereal was promoted as a part of a nutritious breakfast. The only thing you really worried about in food was if it had trans fat. It was a time when *Full House* and *Family Matters* made perfectly acceptable babysitters, and you certainly didn't think about PFAS and phthalates in clothing because helllooo windbreakers. Aside from the *swish-swish* sound windbreakers made when I was walking, one of the most satisfying (and sustainable) parts of my childhood were hand-me-downs. There was nothing better than coming home from school to a big black trash bag full of my older cousin's clothes she had outgrown. Why don't adults pass out hand-me-downs to their friends? Recycling clothes among friends is like participating in a Christmas gift exchange any time of year! It's so fun! Unless none of your friends are your size. Then that could be awkward. But fear not—almost equally exciting as hand-me-down hauls (not quite, but almost) are the thrills of finding amazing deals at thrift stores. Thrift shopping has certainly grown in popularity, and it's no wonder because it's an excellent way to get beautiful clothes for cheap. Unless you live in a big city, in which case I feel bad for you because I went to a Goodwill in Nashville and saw a wool sweater that cost sixty dollars. Sixty dollars for a used wool sweater! The wool must have been shorn from downy yaks tended by traditional Tibetan farmers. There are more high-end brands in big-city thrift stores, but my best treasures have been found at small thrift shops in rural areas.

The key to successful thrifting is consistency and patience. It also doesn't hurt to make friends with the workers so you can tell them what you're looking for and ask that they set it aside for you whenever it comes in. This is the one time I will encourage you to buy donuts. First win the workers over with surprise donuts, then one day you can bring in your homemade sprouted oat energy balls made with locally sourced honey (and donuts, because everyone has to make their own choices). You will be bagging all the best woolen and linen pieces in no time.

Some thrift stores accept volunteers and give a discount in exchange for your time. My mom works at a small thrift shop for two hours on Mondays, and in exchange for her time, they allow her to fill a tote bag for five dollars. She has provided so many clothes for my children (and my friend's children) because every Monday she fills a tote bag with fantastic finds. When I'm done with them, I pass them on to friends who pass them on to friends.

---

5 Best Non-clothing Deals
I've Scored While Thrifting

1. Tons of beautiful, original art for $1 a piece
2. An antique handwoven wool rug for $1
3. Our dining room table for $10
4. An outdoor furniture set for $5
5. A mahogany coffee table for $10 that was still being sold in stores priced at $2,000

Other out-of-the-box ideas for getting good, sustainable clothes are: Host a clothing swap among friends or church members. Search for what you want on Etsy, Poshmark, Facebook Marketplace, or eBay. Hit up estate sales—grannies have awesome wool sweaters and skirts hiding in the back of their closets. I have found so many pieces that were in mint condition that cost me only a few bucks. However, be careful of mothballs. Mothballs contain a toxic pesticide, and when you smell a mothball, you are being exposed to those chemicals. I once purchased a pair of winter boots I didn't realize had absorbed that mothball scent until I was driving along with the heat turned on in my car and caught a whiff of it, and, well, all I can say is I felt quite self-conscious the whole time I was on that playdate with my old-lady mothless boots.

One of the best ways to combat fast fashion in your life is adopting a capsule wardrobe. For this, there is no one-size-fits-all solution (unless your capsule wardrobe consists only of mumus; those really are one size fits all).

As with anything in clothing fashion, a capsule wardrobe can be incredibly expensive, or you could put on your thrifty hat and seek out the best deals. But the idea is that you have a limited number of clothes, all of which are high quality. The best-case scenario is that the clothes are made of high-quality, natural fibers and that each piece is something you truly enjoy wearing. You also want tops and bottoms to be easily interchangeable so you can have an outfit that looks great no matter the combination.

This is certainly easier said than done, but as someone who loves the thrill of the thrifting hunt, I've found that building a full capsule wardrobe over time can be an adventure. It certainly doesn't have to be purchased all at once. The benefits of a capsule wardrobe are numerous. It not only spares you from the stress of having a closet overflowing with clothes you don't like or don't even remember buying but also provides you with an eco-friendly option that saves money in the long run and (this is my favorite) makes deciding what to wear much easier. Remember, the idea is that they are pieces of clothing you love and that go well together no matter how you mix and match them. If you're successful at making a capsule wardrobe, then the decision of what to wear should be easy! It goes without saying that this doesn't mean you have to throw out your favorite shirt or not have a specific outfit for a special occasion, but the less extra you have, the better.

Buying a handmade, tailored piece of clothing would cost a small fortune, but if you're feeling adventurous, you could try making your clothes. (I can see you rolling your eyes at that last sentence.) Fabric is expensive, but at least you get to pick the fabrics you want, the style you want, and the size you need.

Don't forget, when you pursue "crunchier" choices in any of these areas, it doesn't have to be all or nothing. That's just not a realistic expectation for anyone. Look around, take a deep breath, and ask yourself, What is a small, simple change I can make that will make my life a little better?

Where do you like to shop for clothes?

SILKY	SCRUNCHY	REALLY VERY CRUNCHY
Amazon Prime has everything I'll ever need	Thrift stores and boutiques	My children have been wearing the same hand-knit wool sweater for ten years. I simply add rows as they grow taller.

Jason Says ——————————— -<<<<-

Some parts of my life I've been doing the crunchy way by accident for years. Take fast fashion, for example. My sense of fashion came to a halt when I discovered zip-up hoodies and Chacos. And if I want to look nice, I throw on a long sleeve button up and roll up the sleeves if it's too hot out. I don't know if Chacos are considered crunchy (there's room for a good toe splay, right?), but I wear those suckers until the sole is worn down and the straps are frayed. And my shirts? I don't care if they are new. You know what I care about? I want them to fit and *maybe* not look dingy. I feel like we're in an era where just about anything goes when it comes to fashion, so really, you can make your look your own. As for me? If boring-and-slightly-outdoorsy-but-not-pompous-about-it is a look, that's me.

CHAPTER 5

The Basic Needs (Part 2)

5. Sleep

I get a bit depressed when I hear the statistic that we spend a third of our lives in bed. That doesn't feel fair for some reason. It seems like there should be some sort of hack where we could get away with sleeping a lot less. Maybe there is and we don't know it. Legend has it that Leonardo da Vinci slept only a few hours a day by taking a short nap every couple of hours (he clearly was not married and did not have children). Thomas Jefferson, Thomas Edison, and Napoleon Bonaparte also slept very little, but alas, we are mere plebs destined to rely on rest to function properly. When I had my first son, I was told to wake him every two hours to nurse, which would encourage my milk supply as well as stabilize his blood sugar. Some people will say hogwash to this, but I was an anxious first-time mom who wanted to make sure I was "doing everything right." One week into motherhood, I woke to my son crying. I picked him up and carried him to the living room to nurse him. When I walked in, I saw my husband holding our newborn son, and I started crying. "Why are there two of them?"

My husband looked at me with confusion. "Emily, what are you talking about?" I looked down at my son in my arms and realized I had grabbed my pillow and was grasping it like a baby. "So tired I hallucinated" was not a phrase I ever thought I would use to describe a part of my life, but here we are.

Getting good sleep is a huge part of your overall well-being. Want the short answer on how to remove toxins from your life without adding them to your personality? Go to sleep. According to a study about the neuroprotective aspects of sleep, "When sleep is deprived, the active process of the glymphatic system [the system for clearing the body of waste] does not have time to perform that function, so toxins can build up, and the effects will become apparent in cognitive abilities, behavior, and judgment."[1] When we deprive ourselves of sleep, we deprive ourselves of the opportunity to heal, to detox, to give our brains a clean slate for the next day. Countless studies show the benefits of getting a good night's rest, but we don't have to read those to know a good night's sleep feels good.

So what's keeping us from sleeping? Sometimes it's kids, sometimes it's stress, but a lot of times, it's poor sleep hygiene. It's so tempting to stay up and binge-watch your favorite shows or mindlessly scroll, but it's not worth the cost to your sleep. The light given off by your phone, computer, or TV is called blue light. This type of light tricks your brain into thinking it's still daytime and suppresses the production of melatonin, which is the sleepy-time hormone that helps regulate your circadian rhythm and tells your body when to sleep and when to wake. Many experts recommend you stop looking at devices that produce blue light two hours before your target bedtime. Put your phone away and, unless you have a good reason to sleep with it in the same room as you, try to keep your phone out of the bedroom.

Not scrolling on your phone gives you the perfect opportunity to read a book or practice a new skill. If you insist on seeking more passive entertainment in the evenings, you can listen to an audiobook or catch up on some podcasts. I have heard there are some great true crime podcasts out there. I wouldn't know because if I listened to one of those at night, I wouldn't be able to sleep a wink.

If you're looking to take sleep hygiene to the next level, some people use red light bulbs in the evening to encourage their natural sleep cycles to occur. Think of it like getting in touch with our ancestors; they obviously didn't have electricity, so they would use fires or candlelight in the evening. If you want to take it a step further, spending time in the moonlight prompts the natural release of melatonin as well.

Red bulbs and moonlight aside, our bodies were made to work in tune with nature. Getting early morning sunlight on our bodies and faces prompts the natural production of serotonin—the feel-good hormone. It just so happens that serotonin is a precursor to the production of melatonin. So if you want to sleep well, get outside in the morning. Serotonin deficiency is also linked to a variety of disorders, including anxiety, depression, hormonal dysfunction, eating disorders, chronic pain, migraines, and more. Obviously, most of these involve more complex factors than not getting enough sunlight, but it never hurts to make sure you're doing everything you can to support your body's natural processes.

Getting outside in general, no matter what time of day, is so healthy for you. I'm generally very behind on fads and trends. Having an online audience, I try my best to engage with as many comments and messages as possible, but sometimes I have no clue what people are even saying. *Cheugy*, *yeet*, and *rizz* are all examples of slang I've had to look up. But I felt so ahead of the trends when I saw people saying "touch grass." Yes! Please! If we could all get outside and touch some grass (preferably grass that hasn't been treated with any herbicides, insecticides, or colorants), I know we would be better for it.

Here are a few other common practices for encouraging sleep:

- Exercise. It doesn't have to be high intensity or any sort of fancy program, but getting your heart rate up is associated with a better night's sleep.[2]
- Avoid caffeine beyond your morning cup of coffee. Whether you work in an office or from home, many of us have an afternoon slump that is so hard to get past without caffeinating. Drink water, take a break, and step outside for a moment. You've got this!
- Make sure your sleeping environment is comfortable. Get blackout curtains and choose to sleep in the quietest

part of your home. Treat your bed like a sacred place meant only for sleeping so that you don't associate it with anything else.

It's worth mentioning the importance of creating a healthy sleep environment on top of healthy sleep habits. Beds and bedding can be a major source of toxins in your home. Mattresses are often made of polyurethane foam, which consists of petroleum-based "petrochemicals." Petrochemicals off-gas VOCs, which, as I mentioned before, can cause all sorts of health issues, including respiratory distress and asthma. On top of that, companies treat beds, mattress toppers, and pillows with flame retardants, which have been associated with "diabetes, neurobehavioral and developmental disorders, cancer, reproductive health effects and alteration in thyroid function."[3] As with clothes, mattress covers and sheets are often made of polyester and covered in PFAS, phthalates, and formaldehyde to increase waterproofing and decrease wrinkles. Nice way to spend a third of your life, eh? But don't let it keep you up at night.

What can you do about it? On a basic level, ditch polyester bedding, including comforters and throw blankets, and replace everything with a natural material such as cotton or linen. You can usually even find these things at thrift stores if you're unable to purchase them new. If you have a bit of a bigger budget but can't go too crazy, consider buying a mattress topper that is made of natural latex, organic cotton, or wool. If you have massive amounts of money to spend, buy organic cotton everything and an organic wool mattress stitched into an organic cotton cover and send me pictures so I can live vicariously through you. I will say, I recently met a shepherdess, and she told me she has three years' worth of raw wool that I am welcome to. I have been scheming up a way to make my own wool mattress out of it without making my husband think I'm insane. At the very least I'm thinking about taking the down cushions out of my couch because feathers have been poking through and filling the covers with the wool. Is that the kind of thing I should keep to myself?

6. Shelter

My brother lived in a cave once. You read that right: he was a caveman, and until he met a lady and had a baby on the way, he lived outdoors, doing all his cooking over an open fire. My brother, his wife, and their son, Sage Dragon, now live cozily in a beautiful home in Oregon. If I'm really very crunchy, my brother is really very, *very* crunchy. Because of him, a cave home was my idea of the epitome of a crunchy home . . . until I saw one pop up for sale on Zillow not far from where we live. Of course this listing piqued my interest, so I did some digging. Does it count as spelunking if I was exploring the dark side of cave living? I'm sure there are perfectly livable caves, but I discovered living in any random ol' cave has its downsides—namely, mold and the risk of bat diseases. No amount of mold (or bat disease) is a good thing, so caves are out in my book.

As I mentioned earlier, one of the best things you can

do for your shelter is to improve your air quality. But there's more to a home than clean air. What about the makeup of your home? Flooring made of synthetic materials, carpeting, rugs, paints, and mass-produced furniture are all places where potentially hazardous chemicals can hide. These are chemicals such as formaldehyde (a known carcinogen),[4] parabens (linked to hormone and endocrine disruption),[5] PFAS (linked to learning delays in children and increased risk of cancer),[6] PFCs (linked to reproductive issues),[7] VOCs (linked to an increased risk of asthma),[8] and more.

That sounds like some serious consequences for living in a furnished house. Fear not—just because something is "linked to" a health issue doesn't mean it for sure will affect you, especially if you're taking care of your body and doing your best to minimize chemicals in easier areas, like avoiding added fragrances and not microwaving your food in plastic. Also, some companies are getting privy to the demand for less-harmful products. Lowe's and Home Depot no longer sell carpeting that has been treated with PFAS. Where you can, try to choose products that have third-party certifications for being non-toxic, like OEKO-TEX, UL GREENGUARD, FSC, GOTS, and GOLS. But if that's unattainable, secondhand furniture has already off-gassed, so that can be a safer choice than buying some brands new. My couch was a Facebook Marketplace find, and I love it. It's the cleanest (in every sense of the word) one I could find within a three-hour radius.

You can't do everything perfectly in every area. Again, I don't even think you'd want to be perfect. However, it's wise to be aware of all the places toxins can sneak in and potentially wreak havoc on your health. Try your best where you can; don't allow the stress of trying to live a toxin-free life become more harmful than the toxins you are trying to avoid.

If you could have any kind of vacation, what would you choose?

SILKY	SCRUNCHY	REALLY VERY CRUNCHY
An all-inclusive cruise	A beach on Florida's 30A	A hike on the Appalachian Trail

Jason Says ⋘-

Some of you may remember a video we put out about our family going on vacation, and upon entering the apartment, Emily covers her mouth with her hands and yells for the boys to "Get back! There's mold!" This video, believe it or not, was written and filmed while we were waiting to get a new room because of the actual mold we found throughout the apartment. Now, the practical side of me would typically roll my eyes at this and try to convince Emily that we would only be there for a week and that the mold wasn't "that bad." But in this instance, I couldn't do that. The stuff was everywhere. It was crawling out of the vents like Venom looking for a host to latch onto, and it was even worse in the bedrooms. Even I couldn't justify a tough-it-out stance for our toddlers in this case. Would spending a week there have been *that* bad for us? I mean, it was pretty awful, so maybe. But if that stuff is in your home, it's time to take a hard look at your shelter and either get it fixed or rethink some things.

SECTION 3

The Really Very Crunchy Household

CHAPTER 6

When Your Family Isn't Crunchy

As a child of the 1990s, I have a pretty good idea of how I don't want to raise my kids. I don't blame my parents for setting me in front of a television for a large portion of my childhood. I mean, the '90s brought us some epic animated films that instilled within us a spirit of adventure (and anxiety that our parents would die any day now). Not to mention those Nickelodeon kid-themed game shows primed us to become the FOMO, Instagram-envious consumers we are. What millennial hasn't grown up wondering what it feels like to be slimed?

Looking back, I don't know how my parents (in particular, my dad) didn't realize there was something inherently wrong with putting a plastic-wrapped Honey Bun in the microwave for thirty seconds and feeding it to my siblings and me for breakfast, but they didn't know about the negative effects of BPA, phthalates, or heavily processed food. I clearly remember a television ad that encouraged my parents' generation to feed their kids corn syrup because it was a "natural sugar." Sometimes I can't help but cringe thinking about the amount of purple ketchup and the number of Toaster Strudels, Zebra Cakes, and fake-juice Squeezits I have consumed. I really do wonder what's in a Wonder Ball, because I ate so many of them.

I believe most parents are trying to do their best. My parents worked their butts off to provide a better childhood for me than they had growing up. My dad woke up every day at 2:30 a.m. to deliver bread to all the grocery stores and restaurants within a sixty-mile radius, and my mom was the underpaid manager of our town's most popular family-friendly restaurant. They worked hard to make sure I was warm, my belly was full, and I had an endless supply of batteries for my portable CD player.

Dangerous Toys
We Survived from Our Childhood

- **Rollerblade Barbie**—Her rollerblades shot sparks; whose idea was that?
- **Sky Dancers**—You could blind yourself trying to make a fairy fly.
- **Creepy Crawlers**—You could burn yourself *and* melt toxic plastic so you could form it into the shape of bugs.
- **CSI Fingerprint Examination Kit**—You thought you

> were having some innocent fun, but really you were
> breathing in asbestos from the kit's powder.[1]
> - **Moon Shoes**—You could break your ankle just
>   walking around.

They made the best choices they could. We shopped at thrift stores for gently used clothes instead of buying new. Even if sustainability wasn't the driving force behind that choice, I'll give them some crunchy points there. My dad joined the United States Army Reserve and ended up serving in Iraq for almost two years, and during that time my mom ditched our microwave because she read a chain letter about how plants died when they were watered with water that had been microwaved—the kind of letter that said, "If you love your family and friends, you'll send this to two hundred people."

While most everyone is trying their best, not everyone cares about polyfluoroalkyl substances (PFAS), nor do people like it when you start pointing out all the ways they are poisoning themselves and destroying the environment. Whether we are talking about your partner, your parents, or your kids who are preteens and set in their ways, it's unfair to expect them to see things your way right away.

The most important thing for you to remember is to talk to others the way you would want to be talked to. In his famous book *How to Win Friends and Influence People*, Dale Carnegie says, "Success in dealing with people depends on a sympathetic grasp of the other person's viewpoint."[2] If someone has been doing something one way for their entire life and they haven't come to the conclusion that what they are doing isn't necessarily the best, they probably won't like being told that what they are doing isn't necessarily the best. It's important for you to have grace, understanding, and patience for them to come around.

Making healthy choices involves things that every single person does: eating and drinking, using products on their body and in their home, wearing clothes, and sleeping. So, basically every area of life. Brands spend billions of dollars each year to ensure that their customers are loyal and happy. I don't know about you, but I don't have that kind of spare cash to convince my family that they should buy into my lifestyle choices.

It's nearly impossible to embark on the crunchy journey alone if you have a family because your decisions will inevitably affect them. So what do you do? Pick one person at a time to whom you will bring up one concern at a time and, hopefully, some solutions. Obviously it has to be at the right time and not when someone is feeling vulnerable, like when Amy schooled me on the hand soap.

I think the best place to start is with your spouse or whoever you share your living space with. Whatever you do, don't make the same mistake I did and start the conversation with Little Debbie Christmas Tree Cakes—those things have a cult following. Your audience won't care that *artificial flavors* is code for lab-made chemicals with actual names like methyl cyclopentenolone, diacetyl, 2-methoxy-3-methylpyrazine, and benzaldehyde. Christmas Tree Cakes signal the changing seasons and the very joy of Christmas for some people. When you start with Christmas Tree Cakes, you are basically the person who tells children Santa isn't real. We didn't even do Santa with our kids for the very sake of never wanting to be those people. In short, don't start to inspire change with what a person loves most. Unless it's cigarettes—then please convince them that those things are awful.

Hopefully your person is open to listening to what's important to you. You don't have to make all the changes all at once, especially when doing so affects another person. Start with things that make a huge difference with very little sacrifice. For example, filtered water is a hot topic in the crunchy community. The taste of water isn't going to change much based on what filter you choose, so that's an area that won't feel like a huge sacrifice to those around you, but drinking water is an important thing you want to make sure is clean. Scientists have found that around the country, tap water contains tons of yucky contaminants such as plastics, hormones, heavy metals, and pharmaceuticals. Most people would agree that water shouldn't contain those things. Start easy.

A few other changes that might be relatively easy for "your person" to make include:

- Switching to a deodorant that doesn't contain aluminum (not everyone is ready to ditch it altogether and use a little bit of freshly squeezed lime juice—even my husband has his limits)
- Switching from nonstick cookware that has forever chemicals to cast iron or stainless steel
- Swapping conventional laundry detergent for a fragrance-free, dye-free, all-natural laundry detergent

- Replacing inflammatory cooking oils with olive oil, coconut oil, butter, or lard
- Replacing conventional cola with a probiotic cola (yes, it exists), carbonated water, or even (*gasp*) kefir

When people start their crunchy journeys, they often think it's all or nothing right off the bat, but if you've made it this far into the book, you already know that's not true. Adopting a crunchy lifestyle is like working out. You can't wake up and expect to be able to run a marathon if you haven't run a mile since that one time in high school gym class. Starting out, you aim to be able to run a few minutes, then you work your way up. You may never make it to a marathon (or, in this case, being the ultimate crunchy family), but won't you be in better shape than you were before if, in the end, you can run a 5K? You have to realize that everyone is on their own journey, and they don't have the same experiences or convictions that you have. That's okay.

Thankfully, these days there are alternatives to any conventional, mainstream chemically laden product. If there are changes you want to make as a family, start with a simple internet search for "natural alternative to _____." I like to try DIY alternatives using simple ingredients I can pronounce. Sometimes that doesn't work out. My husband doesn't like putting egg whites in his hair because "it doesn't work as well as American Crew," but I searched and found a hair product we were willing to invest in. If you don't have the budget for thirty-dollar hair wax, you can try the egg whites or even sugar water, lemon juice, or beeswax. If those don't work, look for a "regular" product that is fragrance-free. Again, make changes incrementally as they make sense for you and your family.

From my experience, and from talking to friends and reading thousands and thousands of comments on my videos, I have found that spousal confrontation is not the only concern. There's a ton of confrontation between parents and grandparents or extended family pertaining to the topic of kids. I get it—you have standards for your children and convictions on how you want them to be raised and what they should consume. I decided when I was pregnant that it was important for my kids to have a relationship with their grandparents. I didn't have that kind of relationship, and I don't want my kids to miss out on that. As I said before, my parents did their best with me, but I don't want my kids to have the same childhood I had, so I knew I had to set some boundaries.

I started my motherhood journey with a set of lofty ideals, although it really looked like a big list of don'ts, and then I resented when my parents weren't offering to help with my kids as much as I thought they would. I think they may have been scared they were going to make a decision I didn't approve of. There's no room for fear or resentment in a healthy relationship, so I decided I had to pick my battles. What were my top priorities for my family? What was the best we could do with what we had? I knew that I had to prioritize relationships over perfection, so I landed on my two biggest parameters (aside from obvious physical and emotional safety standards): my kids eat real food, and we don't allow excessive screen time. I decided to be lenient on everything else for the sake of my sons having warm relationships with their grandparents.

My parents like to spoil my kids with gum and candy because they don't usually get those things at home. I used to purchase treats I'm okay with and give them to my parents to have on hand. Now my parents are more accustomed to our crunchy ways, and they search out those things on their own. This approach definitely takes more time and effort up front, but remember: you don't become really very crunchy immediately. The more you insist on healthy changes and actively assist in those changes, over time, your wishes (hopefully) will be understood and accepted.

It's up to you to pick what areas are most important to you, make them respectfully known in a kind and gentle yet firm way, and provide adequate resources for people to respect your decision. A healthy lifestyle goal to adhere to is the 80/20 rule. Eighty percent of the time you follow your strict convictions, and 20 percent of the time you let them slide. Living a crunchy life is all about minimizing your toxic load. That said, be mindful of what you're allowing within your 20 percent, as there should be limitations. I'm not sure you could legitimately say that smoking cigarettes when you wake up in the mornings could be considered part of your 20 percent. I'm pretty sure a single cigarette would take up the full 100 percent for your day. But really, just be reasonable with your 20 percent. If you are the gatekeeper to your family's health, you can take solace in the fact that an occasional "exposure" isn't going to be the undoing of your family's wellness.

One such exposure came at the hands of a seemingly innocent but actually nefarious frozen yogurt shop. You know the type of place: The brilliant walls are lined with enough soft-serve machines that no child has to wait in line for their favorite flavor. The colorful buffet of hard candies, gummies, and syrups could rival Willy Wonka's chocolate factory. And there's no way a five-year-old is going to settle on a couple of cookie crumbles or a simple dollop of whipped cream. No. They'll want the lot. It's a crunchy mom's nightmare, but my parents desperately wanted to take the boys. I decided to make an exception to my real-food rule and let them go. Before they left, I said, "Please no candy toppings and no food dye." That evening I asked my then five-year-old if he'd had fun and what flavor he picked.

"Watermelon," he said with wide eyes.

My heart dropped. "What color was it?"

"Red!" he said with such vigor because, of course, his favorite color is red.

In that moment I had to decide how I would handle the situation. I called the dairy wonderland to confirm that my suspicion of red dye, the devil's color, was indeed present. The woman on the phone probably thought I was crazy when I asked her for details about the ingredients of the watermelon "yogurt." "It says red, then the number sign, then forty. Does that tell you anything?"

I had to keep myself from shouting into the phone, "*Yes*, it tells me everything! I have been betrayed! Betrayed, I tell you, by the very people I love the most! This is the worst-case scenario. Don't you know the negative effects of food dye? How dare you serve innocent children such a thing! Especially *red dye*!" Instead, I replied with a "Yes, thank you."

I decided that confronting my parents in anger was not

the best way forward. A shame because I'd devised an elaborate plan that involved inviting them over for dinner where I'd serve them locally sourced organic grass-finished beef burgers on a handcrafted sourdough bun with homemade mayonnaise made with eggs from pasture-raised, herbally managed hens. When my mom asked what she could bring, I'd tell her pickles. She'd show up with her favorite bread-and-butter pickles, and I could casually say, "Oh, Mom, did you know these pickles have food dye? Almost all store-bought pickles do! Just like *watermelon frozen yogurt!*"

Instead, I took a deep breath. This was not my ideal, but it was also not a tragedy. As we do when parenting our children, we should look at those who interact with our kids through a lens that interprets their actions generously. A lot of times people aren't trying to go against our wishes. They truly aren't thinking about all the things we are passionate about, and that's fair. Was the food dye in the frozen yogurt a big deal to me? Yes. But was it worth making my parents feel shame over it? No. In my opinion, showing love and kindness to someone who was not trying to hurt my child was more important than raising a stink about it.

So, what about people who think you're insane and don't care about your wishes? That's a tricky and unfortunate spot to be in. There's not much you can do other than ask them to listen to your concerns. If it were me, I would treat the conversation like I were a prosecutor trying to lay out all the evidence I have against the defendant. Or wait, am I the defendant and they're prosecuting me? Either way, toxins are the guilty party in my mind, and there's a lot of scientific evidence showing the negative effects they have on our bodies. Try avoiding emotionally charged language, and keep the focus on the toxins instead of using "you" language. Depersonalization in any confrontational conversation makes the offender feel better.

A more aggressive conversation could sound something like this:

I'm so tired of you buying mutagenic munchies for our children when you take them to the store. Is it really that hard to avoid buying so much candy?

Maybe a better approach would be:

Hey! I recently read an article from the *International Journal of Occupational and Environmental Health* that said Red No. 3 causes cancer in animals.[3] It has been banned from use in cosmetics but is still used in candies and even maraschino cherries! I was curious, so I checked the Dubble Bubble bag and even it has Red No. 3. Why in the world would the FDA allow a known carcinogen in kids' candy? Crazy! It worries me. You think we could start buying alternatives that don't have dyes just to be safe?

You could also send them a few Really Very Crunchy videos and gauge their reaction. "On a scale of one to ten, how crazy do you think this Emily girl is? One being 'What's funny about this? It's completely normal' and ten being 'I would jump off a bridge if I knew this woman.'" If they are at a ten, then you've got quite the uphill battle on your hands.

Try to be heartfelt and genuine in connecting with whoever you're trying to convince. Don't forget that even the slightest incremental changes matter. Maybe your mom isn't ready to give up her scented plug-ins for herself, but she'd be willing to unplug them the day before your family visits if you tell her that you recently learned they contain hormone disruptors. You can't expect to change everyone's entire lives to suit your justifiable priorities. Remember that little by little, a little becomes a lot. So maybe today it's unplugging the plug-ins, but before you know it, she'll be making simmer pots and burning beeswax candles.

The journey to becoming crunchy starts in your own life. There is power in making positive changes for yourself that people may notice. Some might see the steps you're taking and start asking questions. And if they ask questions, the door is open for a conversation that could change their lives forever and could create a ripple effect that shapes your family and other families for generations to come. That progression of influence can play out even in areas of life that have nothing to do with being crunchy, like faith, relationships, parenting styles, and the breaking of generational cycles. That's what we want to do as humans, right? Don't we all long to be the best version of ourselves that we can?

Whoa. That was deeper than I expected it to be. Just don't forget not to lead with Christmas Tree Cakes, and you'll be fine.

What is your favorite way to unwind with your spouse after a long day?

SILKY	SCRUNCHY	REALLY VERY CRUNCHY
Binge-watch your favorite show	Take a warm Epsom salt bath with soy-wax candles burning	Walk barefoot in the grass while sipping beet juice

Jason Says ⟵⟵⟵

When you live with someone for so long, you start to under-stand what's going on behind their eyes when they look at you. A frown doesn't always mean disapproval, and a smile definitely doesn't always mean they're happy. This was never more true than the time I took our two boys camping while Emily went on a short trip with a friend. I made a Really Very Crunchy video about the experience, and in it, I joke about not being able to start a fire with a flint, so I opted for a lighter and a fire starter log. I remember Emily watching the video and then looking up at me. "Oh, that's funny," she said. "Did you actually use that fire starter?"

"Yes," I replied.

She nodded, smiled, looked at the screen. "And then roasted marshmallows over it?"

I looked from the screen to her smiling face, back to the screen, back to her smiling face.

Her eyes read, "This video is really funny. Good job," but her mind was screaming, "Did you *really* roast marshmallows

over a fire starter log and feed them to my babies? Do you
know the kind of chemicals a fire starter gives off?"

All that to say: Emily practices what she preaches. She
could have called me an idiot and rattled off all the ways I was
causing incurable diseases in our children, which would have
been grounds for a long argument. Instead, I got the subtle
message that maybe next time I should just use a match and
some dried leaves for the fire, because honestly, I had never
thought about the chemical makeup of a fire starter log. And
guys, it's really not great...

CHAPTER 7

❧

What Crunchiness Means for Friendships

Let's be honest, being crunchy can make things awkward. Before you know it, you're that weird lady who's not wearing shoes to an event (indoor or outdoor) and is offering people raw carrots for aiding in estrogen detoxing. If they won't take the carrots, maybe you persuade them to eat special chocolate to detox parasites, or maybe you ask them how their gut microbiome is doing. These things are conversation starters no matter who you are, but they may not be the spark that ignites a lasting friendship.

Listen: friendships are hard, especially when you're already awkward, and being crunchy only adds to that awkwardness. If you've watched my videos over the last couple of years, you've probably seen that every now and then I'll post one about trying to make a new friend at the park or working my way into a group of moms who are talking about a television show their children watch, and it leaves the viewer cringing and laughing with me. (With me, right? Right?) Well, those videos are closer to the "real me" than any other videos I post, so if you're hoping to read this chapter to learn how to make friends, sorry to disappoint. My only advice there is to be kind, be genuine, and show up . . . and then keep showing up. It's worth pushing through those awkward times.

Differences in parenting choices also add to the awkwardness. In my experience, (but not in my opinion) it matters to some people what material your kids poop in, where and how they go to sleep, how much screen time you allow, and what kinds of snacks you feed your kids.

If you've had babies or plan to have babies, you know that the baby phase can be both the sweetest and one of the most difficult seasons you will face in your lifetime. I never understood why sleep deprivation was used as a form of torture until I had a baby. In my extremely sleep-deprived moments, an interrogator could have gotten anything out of me. "Yes, okay, I cheated my way through geometry in high school by copying off my crush's homework and watching him for all the answers on tests. ('Touch your forehead for A, your nose for B, and your chin for C.') If I could go back, I wouldn't do that!"

Jason and I had friends whose baby was a year older than ours, so naturally, they had everything figured out ahead of time and were ready to let us in on all the secrets and tricks they learned in their first year. That's what friends are for!

You can understand the look of shock on my face when they told me that when he was around six months old, they closed their child in his room at night and let him scream until he threw up. "He sleeps great on his own now!" I know, I know, that's extreme and not the case for everyone as there are different levels of "sleep training." Don't get all bent out of shape if you think I'm coming at you—I'm not.

Not wanting to create a rift in our friendship, I took a deep breath and nodded, knowing I wouldn't be able to take their advice on getting our child to sleep. Jason and I talked about it, weighed what they had to say, and knew it wasn't the route we wanted to go for our children. And things would have been fine if we could have left it at that. But weeks and months went by. My son wasn't a good sleeper even though I tried my best to follow schedules and cycles and advice from books that promised sleep. Things weren't good. I felt like I was failing as a mother. We were all tired. Jason and I fought over little things that didn't matter. Neither one of us was in a great place emotionally, mentally, or physically. Worse still, we didn't have support.

Instead of our friends accepting the fact that we were doing things differently and making space for that, the opposite happened. Time after time the mom would reach out to me to say how well her son was sleeping and how rested she felt. I could be talking to someone about the farmers market on Saturday, and she would walk up and say, "Jaxson's been sleeping like a champ this week! I've never felt so good!" (No, his real name isn't Jaxson.) And then she would give me a side glance as if to say, "You should take my advice. Your life would be better. Come over to my side. The water's fine!"

It made me feel small. As though every time we hung out, I was going to be told by my friend that I was doing something wrong and that I was a bad mom for continuing to do it. I still don't know what her motivation was for doing that, but it hurt our friendship. Though it's not something I dwell on anymore and we've all moved on, the friendship never truly mended. They have wonderful, happy kids, and both of my kids now sleep great through the night. Turns out, every child is different. We bedshared from the beginning with my second son and never once tried to schedule anything, and he was a champion sleeper. (Except for in the car. Why won't my kids sleep in the car?)

What I have come to learn is that you need to surround yourself with people who will support you, even if you aren't doing things exactly the same way they do them. At the same time, you need to be that friend for others, even if they aren't doing things the way you think is best. I imagine she and I would still be friends today if, instead of giving me a report on her child's sleep every week, she would have come up to me, given me a hug, and said she was praying for me and that she was there to talk if I ever needed it.

In an ideal world, there would be no conflict among friends for different parenting choices, and our babies would sleep through the night starting from day one. But that's not how life works, and it is our job to make the best of these times. Just know that sometimes doing what's best for *your* nest can lead to some uncomfortable interactions, and that's normal.

When you're on a crunchy journey, people around you aren't always going to understand what you're doing or why you're doing it. Many people have never given a second thought to the chemical makeup of Doritos. Most people don't think about EMFs from baby monitors or proper foot health. It's not our job to convert them. Crunchiness is about you trying to make healthier choices for your life, not someone else's. We all know the mantra by now, right? Let's say it together: *crunchy is a spectrum.* It is a choice you make in various scenarios. You may be crunchy in some cases but not in others. And that's okay.

I think the urge to preach the crunchy lifestyle has to do with the expectations we set for ourselves and the fact that, sometimes, the pursuit of crunchiness requires us to take a much more difficult path than the one others are on. Let's face it, having a Nutri-Grain bar is a lot easier than making your own version of a granola bar. It's easier to set a child in front of a screen than it is to encourage them to explore imaginative play or to read them book after book after book. It's easier to spend most of your hours indoors with a bunch of gadgets than it is to go outside no matter the weather and enjoy the fresh air. And when you recognize that the path you have chosen is harder than a lot of other people's, jealousy can creep into your mind and make a home. That's when the air of superiority comes in and you feel the need to convert others to the way you're doing things, especially when they are already your friends. Don't do it.

Here's a hard-and-fast rule I've adopted. Unless someone asks me for tips or suggestions on ways to improve their life or their health, I try not to mention my crunchy approach to life except to share about me or my family, and only if it's a natural part of the conversation. Take, for example, Father's Day. I made two versions of banana pudding—one for my family and one for my dad. He doesn't care about all the junk that's in boxed pudding; he wants it to taste like his favorite memories of eating pudding. I'm not going to shame him for eating it, but I'm also not going to feed the boxed pudding to my kids. End of story.

Of course, you may think that's rich of me to say since I have a social media account wholly dedicated to crunchy comedy. But hopefully you see that for what it is: a lighthearted approach to making crunchy funny. Because, honestly, there's a lot to laugh about in the crunchy space, no matter what side you fall on.

It's difficult not to come across as judgy when you are in social situations that require you to take a stand for your lifestyle. This is particularly true in parenting. My first viral video was "Crunchy Mom at a Birthday Party." It was written and shot to be a crunchy mom doing her best, not to come across as judgy and completely failing. Lo and behold, a couple of months later, my two children and I were invited to a party at a skating rink where cake was provided by the skating rink. Skating rink cake—those words haunted me. I had grown up going to that skating rink. I knew what kind of cake they would be serving, and I knew it would include *all* the things, including dyes, seed oils, refined sugar, and grains. I know it's fine to indulge every once in a while, but I also know (from experience) those kinds of things generally make my kids feel terrible.

I try to make sure I'm not scaring my kids away from food. I don't want them to be afraid of eating something just because I don't think it's a healthy choice. That's a recipe for an eating disorder. It is not a child's job to worry about food. I want my kids to be thinking about having fun, not about the dangers lurking in sheet cake. And I certainly don't want to make them feel excluded.

I did my cake-choice spiel the day before, and the boys chose homemade. The skating rink was a sensory overload, and the music was so loud it was next to impossible to hear what was going on at the party table. So when the cake was served, I pulled out the glass container with two frosted, naturally dyed cupcakes and set them in front of my boys, and no one seemed to care or even notice. I didn't make a show about it. And when my boys ended up wanting some skating rink pizza, I pretended I couldn't hear them because it was so loud. I'm kidding. I smiled and nodded and let them have a slice—no need to make a scene.

I was grateful to my friend who was hosting the party, as she knows all about my social media account and, for some inexplicable reason, is still my friend. It's possible to have friends who don't agree with you, but you love each other just the same. She said "no gifts" for the party. That seems crazy to me; a birthday party without gifts? But I respected her choice and didn't bring a gift. Give-and-take, mutual respect, doing everything with a heart of kindness and understanding—that's what friendship is about.

There are many variables that could cause an awkward situation, but it's best to be up front with people, if possible, rather than take them by surprise in the moment. No matter what, if you stick to your guns on every issue, you will run into awkward situations, and navigating them can be tricky. Sometimes you're going to fail. Sometimes you'll be rejected.

But remember that life is about balance, and you have to decide what your boundaries are as well as what you're willing to compromise on. Where *can* you be flexible?

I have a bit in my videos where I play the part of a "silky" mom. As with everything on my account, it's meant to make people laugh and not meant to judge anyone, as I make fun of crunchy moms and silky moms alike. This mom has been dubbed by the fans as the "Coke-shirt mom" because every time I portray this character, I'm wearing a T-shirt given to my husband for his birthday one year by his brother. This character is the antithesis of the crunchy mom character. She yells for the kids to get up for school so they don't miss the bus. She promises to buy them more Skittles for their school lunches. She tells them that if the bully at school messes with them again, they should "sock 'em in the face like I taught ya!"

In one video, the crunchy mom and the Coke-shirt mom meet each other at the park. As they watch their kids play, they make snide remarks to each other, indicating that their way of life is far superior to the other's, until their kids collide with each other and both moms have the exact same reaction to make sure their kids are okay. When I wrote the skit, I didn't even anticipate the message that would come forth from the editing. It turned out to be much sweeter than I expected. It showed that the crunchy mom and the Coke-shirt mom could find a middle ground—that there didn't need to be judgment between them. We all love our kids, and we want what's best for them. Let's lift one another up and encourage one another because we are all on this journey called life, and that journey looks different for each and every one of us.

*Friends are coming from out of town. What will you do
to entertain them?*

SILKY	SCRUNCHY	REALLY VERY CRUNCHY
Mario Kart party	Rent bikes and ride around town	Hit up the farmers market and prepare a meal with your finds

Jason Says ———————————— -«««-

For some reason, I've always been able to talk to older people better than I can talk to my peers. When you talk to your peers, everything has to be surface level, at least at first. You've got to tiptoe around certain subjects, and this is especially true about parenting. But when you talk to old people, they don't care. Your kid runs out of the house naked because he needs you to help him wipe poop off his butt? Old people don't care. Their kids did it. Their grandkids do it.

"You sleep train? Don't sleep train? Whatever, man. Do your thing. My kids are grown up and doing fine, except Jimmy's still in prison, and I'm happy to talk about that too."

A couple of our dearest friends live in Washington and are now in their eighties. We met them on a cruise ship from England to Florida (a cruise home was cheaper than a flight), and they are a delight. They have nothing to prove, nothing to judge you for. Our kids are younger than their grandkids, and they have been witness to all walks of life. They are the kind of friends I want to be to my peers and that I hope my peers will be to me.

CHAPTER 8

Making Crunchy Kids

Pregnancy

I have shared many early forays into my crunchy life, but my *real* crunchy journey began after I had my first son. It's fairly common for crunchy moms to admit they became crunchy when they were suddenly responsible for making decisions that affected the health and longevity of another human being. Did you know that if a baby is inadequately nourished in the womb, it can lead to increased risks of developing childhood and adult chronic diseases?[1] No pressure though. It is mind-blowing to me that the first thousand days of life, the time spanning roughly between conception and one's second birthday, is when the foundations of optimum health, growth, and neurodevelopment across the life span are established.[2] Across the life span! That itty-bitty baby does not have the ability to make its own decisions that can impact it forever. That's a huge job.

Talking about anything related to parenting is a touchy subject. It's basically impossible to go through the baby years without offending someone. "Oh, you're nursing? Well, you'd better cover up!" "Oh, you're giving your baby a bottle? Don't you know what boobs were made for?" You can never do everything right because there is no right for everyone. I think the question you should ask yourself is: What is the best I can do in the position I'm in? Crunchy is a spectrum, and it doesn't look the same for everyone. Also, understand that not all moms can (or want to) stay home with their kids. This obviously influences certain crunch-level decisions. Crunchy parenting should never be about making the wrong choice. It's about you making the right choices for your family.

Parenting Choices
I've Made That Someone Felt the Need to Negatively Comment On

- Not putting socks on my infant . . . in July
- Letting my kids get a cookie at the bakery . . . just not one with dye
- Letting my kids cut things in the kitchen . . . with a butter knife
- Letting my toddler climb the stairs on a playground . . . while I watched from a few feet away
- "Publicly" nursing my son . . . alone in our car

No matter your situation, some of the best advice for growing and bringing up babies is to be anxious for nothing.[3]

Try not to stress. Mounting evidence shows that prenatal maternal stress affects the brain and behavior of her offspring.[4] Had someone told me this when I was pregnant, I probably would've replied, "Okay, don't think about elephants!" It's nearly impossible. But I also probably would've taken steps to decrease my stress. Like not moving two times in one pregnancy. Or not switching jobs during pregnancy. Or not googling so many questions. As someone who has struggled with worrying her entire life, I know it's hard to let go of, especially when you want to do your best. But one of the crunchiest things you can do is to figure out a way to decrease your anxiety. It's not just for your baby but for you too! Be intentional; be informed.

With so many things to be anxious about, I find one way to decrease anxiety is to make informed decisions. Don't float through pregnancy and motherhood reacting to situations as they come up. Have a plan to keep yourself from being reactive. The internet is a beautiful and terrifying place—things can get weird really quick. Like when I was researching baby resilience and learned that babies and children can regrow their fingertips until the age of eight. That fact, while cool, grosses me out and isn't the type of resilience I was looking for. Avoid falling into too many rabbit holes. Get advice from real moms, midwives, doctors, and doulas you trust. Use their advice and do some online searching of pros and cons on their stance. If you're about to be a first-time mom, or know a first-time mom, here's a list of could-be-anxiety-inducing topics that you can calmly approach and make informed decisions about:

1. **Healthy pregnancy nutrition**—Turns out maybe you shouldn't eat a whole pizza twice a week. Having a healthy, balanced diet in pregnancy can be a contributing factor to your birth goals. Look into different types of pregnancy nutrition, and choose what's right for you. Some diets to consider include Ayurvedic, Weston A. Price, and a general holistic pregnancy approach.

2. **Pelvic floor education and exercises**—Remember how your mom said she couldn't jump on a trampoline or she'd pee herself? That doesn't necessarily have to be your fate.

3. **Effects of epidural use**—Some risks of epidural use include slowing or stopping of labor, less effective pushing, increased interventions, and disruption of maternal bonding.[5]

4. **Natural pain management practices for labor**—If the risks of epidural use don't sound worth it to you there are options for managing pain or discomfort in childbirth. These include but aren't limited to meditation, breathing exercises, massage, water therapy, and visualization.

5. **Benefits of delayed cord clamping**—According to the American College of Obstetricians and Gynecologists, "Delayed umbilical cord clamping increases hemoglobin levels at birth and improves iron stores in the first several months of life, which may have a favorable effect on developmental outcomes."[6]

6. **To circumcise or not to circumcise**—If you're having a hospital birth in the United States, make this decision

before you go. It is not something you should decide in the bleary-eyed moments of being postpartum.

7. **Vaginal swabbing in case of C-section**—Babies born via C-section are at a greater risk of developing immune and metabolic disorders, but exposing them to their mother's vaginal fluid may help increase their microbiome diversity to be similar to that of a vaginally born baby.[7]

8. **The golden hour for babies**—The benefits of skin-to-skin contact for baby and mother are immense if it's done for one hour immediately after birth without interruptions.

9. **Benefits of kangaroo care**—The benefits of skin-to-skin contact from mother and father continue for several months, so this kind of closeness should be squeezed in whenever possible.

10. **Benefits of colostrum**—Even if you plan to formula feed, breastfeeding your baby a couple of times may be worth it since colostrum is full of antibodies, nutrients, and antioxidants that lay a strong foundation for your baby's immune system and wellness.

The choices you make are no one's business, so don't feel the need to justify them if they are different from the choices of those around you. The most important thing is that you arm yourself with information so you can make the best decisions for you. If that means you want an epidural after you've researched it, that's your choice. Don't forget that pregnancy, labor, and delivery are challenging and intense experiences, so have grace for yourself. Making informed decisions about your ideal plans is great, but it's crucial to hold your plans loosely so that you can accept whatever happens. With both of my pregnancies I had some medical complications and ended up having to be induced. While I chose to forgo an epidural with my second, it wasn't the at-home, beeswax candle lit, completely natural birth I envision when I talk about natural births. When your expectations and reality don't line up, it can be hurtful and even traumatic. Those early days are so short, and if things don't go exactly as you wished, that doesn't mean you can't have a wonderful, meaningful relationship with your child. Don't allow yourself to get so stuck on certain aspects of birth and even the early days of motherhood that you lose perspective. I urge you to find healing. You are here right now; now is what matters. That goes for your entire parenting journey.

Babywearing

When my first son was born, my husband was working at a local newspaper for barely above minimum wage. I was a nanny. We didn't have a lot of money. I followed a lot of accounts on Instagram that made having a newborn look aesthetically pleasing. Read: rattan everything, organic cotton in neutral colors, and husbands who seemed to have an endless supply of paternity leave. We didn't have the funds for anything rattan or organic cotton, and my husband hadn't even worked at his job long enough to have vacation days, so he used his two sick days as his paternity leave. I went back to nannying after two weeks because we needed the money. I'm thankful for this period of time because not having money opened my eyes to all the unnecessary items that are pushed onto unsuspecting parents. Working outside my own home, I had to figure out how to streamline caring for my baby without transporting a swing, a bouncer, a Bumbo, a skidder-mer-inki-dinki-dink, or whatever the latest must-have baby container is called.

A lot of my crunchy choices were made from logic. For example, the baby carrier. A baby carrier was life changing for me. I could keep my little baby tucked close and have my hands free to help the other child I was caring for. I could breastfeed in the carrier, and my little one loved napping there too. I think I might have used a stroller once or twice the entire time my boys were "stroller age," as it didn't make sense to me to have to lug around a giant expensive contraption when all I needed was a simple piece of cloth. I always thought it was comical when a veteran mom stopped me at the store or a park to comment on how they didn't have stuff like carriers when she was a mom of littles. But they did! Baby wearing is centuries old, and while the art lost popularity, it is making a resurgence with the knowledge that baby wearing has many benefits. Research suggests a link between proper baby wearing and good developmental hip health. Research also suggests baby wearing is beneficial for emotional and intellectual growth because frequent physical contact with a caregiver promotes attachment and bonding.[8] Of course, anything can be done wrong, so it's important to look up the correct, safe way to wear your baby. Babies can't live their entire infancy in a carrier. Crunchy and conventional parenting experts will tell you it's important to put babies in a safe spot on the floor and give them the ability to move freely. This prevents flat spots on their heads, strengthens neck and shoulder muscles, and improves babies' motor skills. Like the excessive use of television or screens with young children takes away opportunities for free play and exploration, when you bind, prop, or buckle a baby into a container, you take away an opportunity for development. It's not entirely up to the parent; obviously other factors influence development, but parents and caregivers do play an extremely important role in maximizing their child's potential and can "make it or break it," so to speak.

Moms can sympathize with me here, but I can't read the poem "Babies Don't Keep" without bursting into tears. Babies are babies for such a short time. That time is full of intense learning and emotions, but when you put it into perspective, that time is so short. At the risk of sounding cliché, try your best to soak it all in, savor it.

Bedsharing

As I mentioned, we struggled with sleep with my first son. I tried to follow all the "rules" and schedules and eat-wake-sleep cycles, but he had different plans. When I stopped reading books and started reading my baby's cues, everything got easier and more enjoyable. I was so gung ho about getting my baby to sleep in a crib that I wasn't getting any sleep myself. About six months in, I decided to forget the whole crib situation and embrace what my baby wanted, which was to be near me. A baby's need for comfort and connection is as legitimate of a need as warmth or food. I decided to start bedsharing, and it was the best thing I could have done for my baby and for my sleep (just as there are safe crib practices, there are safe cosleeping practices that should be followed).

Sometimes cosleeping looks weird on the outside. If anyone had asked for a tour of our home, at one point they would have noticed we had two queen beds pushed together, which we called our megabed. I need space when I sleep, but I still wanted to be in the same room as my husband. I will never be able to relate to those people who can sleep spooned up close to another person. That is not me. In fact, here's a little marriage tip: if someone is always stealing the blanket, stop sharing blankets. You can just stack them when you make the bed. Problem solved. When baby number two came along, we needed even more space, so we had two queen beds and a full-size bed all pushed together—we called that our ultra-megabed. Our toddler loved jumping around on it. Our room was literally a bed-room. I even tried making it aesthetically pleasing when I purchased two twin headboards off Facebook Marketplace and butted those on either side of our queen headboard. I also found two matching king-size quilts at a salvage store that could cover the entire bed. It didn't work. It looked like three different headboards awkwardly positioned behind three different beds with two different quilts spread across it. If there's one thing I've learned from being me, there's no hiding awkward. I just have to embrace it.

I think couples fear that their marriage will suffer with

cosleeping because they won't have sex. Psst, there's more than one place to have sex. Making your relationship healthy and a priority doesn't hinge on sleeping on the same mattress at night. But, again, every family is different, and you have to do what's best for you. Nothing you choose has to be forever; it's a healthy practice as a family to look at your habits every month or so and evaluate what's working for you and what's not. If you decide a decision isn't serving you, it's okay to change your mind, even if you were passionate about making a change in that area.

Nutrition

Nutrition is an extremely sensitive topic, so I hope you can understand I'm writing about this subject with the understanding that our bodies fail us. This is an imperfect world, and some things are out of our control. Truthfully, natural-minded people are going to lean toward the most natural choice. So if you're medically able to breastfeed and are nourishing your body well enough to produce enough milk and are mentally in a good place, and you have the option between formula and breastfeeding, I would highly recommend breastfeeding. That sounds like an awful lot of caveats, and it is because everyone's situation is different. The American Academy of Pediatrics (AAP), the American Medical Association (AMA), and the World Health Organization (WHO) all recommend breastfeeding as the best choice for babies. It is not always easy; there will be times you're so swollen with milk that Dolly Parton herself would congratulate you on your bosom. You might lose enough feeling in the areola region that you won't notice your boob hanging out when you open the door to get the package from the mail lady (poor gal changed her route because of it—she blamed her ankle, but I know the truth). Or you might lose some sleep because breast milk is more easily digested, meaning the baby gets hungry faster. It's perfectly normal for breastfed babies to wake every two to four hours for the first six months of their life (and beyond, depending on the kid).

All those inconveniences seem worthwhile, though, when you consider that breastfeeding helps protect babies from a variety of infections, meningitis, allergies, asthma, diabetes, obesity, and sudden infant death syndrome (SIDS). Chemicals in your baby's saliva provide feedback to your body to change the makeup of your milk to meet your baby's needs as it grows. Breastfeeding is truly an amazing miracle—it reduces a mom's risk of certain kinds of cancer, and best of all, it's absolutely free!

Obviously, as I mentioned before, there are lots caveats to nursing. Not all women can breastfeed for one reason or another. If you were one of those people and you wanted to breastfeed but couldn't, I'm so sorry. Formula absolutely does provide the nutrients babies need to grow and thrive. I tried finding that ever-elusive scientific study that was likely passed through a chain email of 1990s crunchy moms about how babies who nursed grow up to have higher IQs than those who were formula fed, and it doesn't exist. Formula feeding your baby does not mean your baby won't grow and thrive and laugh and be just as smart as any other baby. Some moms worry they won't be as bonded to their baby if they use a bottle, but the important thing is your presence. Looking into your baby's eyes and holding them close—these are the things that deepen your relationship with your baby, not the vessel in which the milk flows forth.

Formula feeding does have a couple of potential downsides. It might mean your child will be at a higher risk for developing asthma and allergies,[9] but those things can depend on a variety of circumstances, like genetics and environmental factors. Studies also suggest formula-fed babies are more likely to become picky eaters,[10] which can be a tricky thing to overcome. If breastfeeding isn't in the cards for you, focus on getting (or making) the highest-quality formula you can. Just because it says "organic" doesn't mean it isn't highly processed and full of sweeteners. The most popular formula sold is made of nearly 50 percent corn syrup, followed by soy, seed oils, and more sugar. The first two ingredients come from corn and soy, both of which are largely GMO crops that are heavily sprayed with the herbicide glyphosate, which has been deemed as "probably carcinogenic to humans."[11]

Soon enough, babies start showing an interest in food other than milk, and this is another opportunity for you to be informed. First foods are exciting! Also, can we all agree that it is time for the rice cereal and banana mush narrative to change? If the idea of eating a certain food makes you gag, it is worth considering why we'd offer it to our babies. Feed them yummy stuff! Some of my favorite options for a baby include soft-boiled egg yolk, bone marrow with whipped butter, and liver pâté. Okay, maybe those want to make you gag too, but in this case it doesn't mean they aren't excellent options. None of these foods were recommended to me by a pediatrician or veteran mom, but these are well known to be nutrient dense and easily accessible foods. My favorite website for learning about setting a solid foundation for your child to enjoy all types of foods is solidstarts.com.

I believe parents set up their kids for pickiness by making a few mistakes early on. One is introducing sweet foods too soon. It's not just the obvious stuff either—popular baby food brands, such as Gerber, use "fruit juice concentrate" as a nice-sounding way of adding sugar to baby food. Added sugars are everywhere; it's no wonder toddlers these days are consuming upward of seventeen teaspoons of sugar each day.[12] The recommended amount for children ages two to twelve is less than six teaspoons.[13] Worldwide we are becoming less and less healthy as more and more sugar is introduced into our diets.

Parents lay the foundation for their child's lifelong relationship with food. Kids are funny and always trying to figure out the world by testing boundaries. Maybe you've done everything right. Maybe you even fed them liver pâté as their first food. They might still have a meltdown over green beans. Even if your kid hates a food at first, don't give up. Keep offering it in different ways. My favorite book on raising a non-picky eater is *French Kids Eat Everything*. In the book, Karen Le Billon suggests offering kids food with the caveat "you don't have to like it, but you do have to taste it."[14] You won't convince kids to like certain foods by forcing them. But you also won't get kids to have a varied palate by offering Nature Valley candy—I mean, granola bars—when they don't eat their dinner.

Everyone Poops, **Especially Babies**

Diapers are gross. I'm not just saying that for the obvious reasons. Diapers are treated with and made of potentially hazardous chemicals,[15] plus disposable diapers are estimated to take about 450 years to decompose, so all the disposable diapers that have ever been created and pooped in are still in existence. That's a disgusting thought. The more eco-friendly and healthier option is cloth diapers. But have you considered that there's something even better than that? Two words: elimination communication. Babies can learn to go to the potty starting at a very young age. Just as they can communicate their need to eat or their need for comfort, they can let us know they need to use the potty if we are adept at reading their cues. My younger son started pooping on the potty when he was five months old. Elimination communication is incredibly empowering for children. It teaches them independence over something they can control at a young age. It also encourages self-confidence.

If you're looking for great information on elimination communication, check out godiaperfree.com.

Entertainment

Any crunchy mom will tell you there are two things you should avoid giving your kids for as long as possible: one we've already touched on, and that's refined sugar. The second is screen time. Well, and shoes, but that's more debatable and we'll touch on that again later. "Sugar and Screens" sounds like it could be a toddler rock song about taking a dangerous path early in life, "Highway to Hell" style. Both sugar and screens are highly addictive; we're talking cocaine-level addictiveness. But their overuse has become so mainstream in our society that no one bats an eye at babies in car seats with tablets propped in their laps or little ones at a restaurant unable to sit still without a snack of fruit chews and their own personal tablet. It's not the parents' fault entirely. I've been in a code-red restaurant situation where my three-year-old was clearly unable to access his prefrontal cortex, the part of the brain responsible for rational decision-making and impulse control. He was flailing, flopping, and flagrantly bellowing his afflictions for the whole flood of fellow patrons to observe. It was embarrassing, humbling, and isolating.

I get it—it's easier. Kids can be coaxed into sitting down and being quiet and not making any messes when they are pacified with screens or sugar. But I wonder whether as a culture we discover the ease of pacification and then rely on it too much. Parenthood can be challenging, and I know what it's like to feel like you're just treading water, just trying to survive. But at what cost? The AAP recommends children ages two and under don't receive *any* screen time or consume *any* added sugar, for good reasons.

Studies link the overuse of screens to speech delays, poor sleep habits, and poor social skills. When parents become reliant on sticking littles in front of screens, they rob their toddlers of opportunities to develop their attention spans, gross and fine motor skills, and impulse control. Most importantly, screens take away opportunities for little ones to engage in imaginative play. Many experts argue that the best learning happens for kids ages five and under when they are engaged in play. The AAP states, "Play allows children to use their creativity while developing their imagination, dexterity, and physical, cognitive, and emotional strength. Play is important to healthy brain development."[16] Nowhere will you read that screens are important to healthy brain development; you'll read the opposite. I'll touch more on screens and the importance of play in the next chapter, but toddlers who don't start out with constant entertainment have an easier time learning to cope with boredom. People often ask me how I'm able to write so many videos and a book and still homeschool and make healthy meals. I'm not a supermom. I fail often, and my house is messy, though I prefer to call it "lived in." But what I do have are a couple of kids who know how to play. You know how moms revel in the peace and freedom that come from nap time? Allow your kids the opportunity to learn how to engage in independent play and you'll never feel desperate for nap time again.

I have tried to keep our toys open ended, like blocks, play silks, a dollhouse, and animal figurines. It's tempting to reach for the flashy light up toys with fun sound effects that draw kids in with their hypnotizing lure. There's nothing inherently wrong about these toys aside from the torture of having to listen to the same song five thousand times, but these kinds of toys are toy-led, they determine how your child plays instead of letting your child decide. Open-ended toys can be played with in a variety of ways—there's no right way to play, and it's up to the child to determine how to use them. They are 90 percent child, 10 percent toy. What I love about open-ended toys is that they foster creativity, problem-solving, and critical thinking. It's one more positive way to allow your child's brain to develop.

Shoes

Everything is cuter in miniature. I mean, have you seen a Shetland pony? This includes teeny tiny shoes, and though Shetland ponies may require tiny horseshoes, the same cannot be said for our children. Allowing children to go barefoot allows thousands of nerves to receive stimulation in the feet. Stimulation means opportunities for neural connections, which means brain growth, development, and learning! Letting your kids go barefoot might just be the easiest and cheapest crunchy decision you can make. Angela Hanscom, a pediatric occupational therapist and author of the book *Balanced and Barefoot*, suggests children should be barefoot as much as possible, "Walking outdoors offers natural messages to children's feet as they walk on different-sized pebbles and uneven ground. The resistance and inconsistency nature offers integrates reflexes in the foot and forms strong arches. Going barefoot out in nature helps to develop normal gait patterns, balance and tolerance of touch in the feet, all of which provide a strong foundation for confident and fluid movement."[17] Going barefoot both inside and outside improves agility and promotes spatial awareness. Unrestricted, natural movement allows kids' feet to develop as they were meant to. The biggest downside to letting your little ones go barefoot is the droves of old ladies who will question your decision. "Where are that baby's socks! Get that baby some shoes!" Ma'am, it's ninety-seven degrees outside—no one needs socks right now.

If you're in a place where your kids do need to wear shoes, say, at the park where there's rubber mulch—hello, heavy metals—or in a public place because who knows what they use to clean those floors, then look for shoes that have a soft, flexible bottom and wide toe box. These kinds of shoes are often referred to as barefoot shoes. I have a list of my favorite brands listed in the resource section at the end of this book. Feet can still reap all the benefits of being barefoot with the proper footwear. But please, for heaven's sake, barefoot shoes or not, take your shoes off when you go home. Shoes worn in public are covered with pesticides, fecal matter, and other toxic chemicals that you bring into your home when you wear your shoes inside.

Crunchy Where It Counts

The cool thing about babies and children is that they are incredibly resilient. Mistakes can be made, choices can be made and changed and changed again, and babies can still turn into emotionally and physically healthy children. More than eating the "right" foods or wearing the "right" shoes or picking the "right" toys, the best possible investment you can make in raising your child isn't even something that can be labeled crunchy, it's time spent together. Spend as much uninterrupted time as you can being fully present with your kids. Not just time spent in the same room as one another but time looking one another in the eyeballs, talking to one another, doing things that deepen your relationship with one another. When you spend time with your kids, you learn so much. Plus, kids are far more likely to listen to and cooperate with a parent who has filled their need for attention and belonging.

I made a video about how geese flying in formation honk to encourage one another to keep up their speed. This video showed me honking at a flock flying over my home. While a lot of my videos are exaggerations of reality or scenarios that happen in my brain, I will admit I do honk at geese. I don't use a duck call or anything, but I do excitedly yell "Honk!" as my boys bounce up and down, honking right along with me. On a scale of mainstream to homeschooled, I'd say our homeschooled-ness shows a bit here, but there is something so exciting about a moment out of your control sneaking up on you and you having a way to celebrate it. I want to infuse my kids' lives with moments that feel meaningful and connected, a feeling they can carry with them as they grow. We also shout "Water tower!" anytime we see a water tower when we are driving. It sounds so silly, but it's a way of creating a sense of belonging, and we all know the drill of shouting it out when we see one.

Some people are fine with being a family by proximity and genetics, but I want more. I want true connection with my kids. Honking at geese is not the only way to make that happen, but the only way your family can have your own "special thing" is if you make it happen.

What's a toddler's happy place?

SILKY	SCRUNCHY	REALLY VERY CRUNCHY
Watching Cocomelon	Riding their balance bike	Making mud pies

Jason Says ────────────── -◀◀◀-

It's four o'clock in the morning, and I've got my headphones on. This morning I'm watching *There Will Be Blood*. Daniel Day-Lewis is incredible, but I think tomorrow when I'm inevitably up at four in the morning, I'm going to watch something a bit lighter. Maybe *Comedians in Cars Getting Coffee*. I look down at our infant in my arms to make sure the phone screen is tilted away from him and that the phone is in airplane mode. He's sound asleep as I rock him. I hope Emily is able to rest until I have to get ready for work.

It's easy to feel completely inadequate as a dad of a newborn. If the mom is nursing and cosleeping, it can feel like the bulk of what you're doing as a dad is watching things happen. But after two babies, I've learned that the ways you can help will depend on the baby and the overall structure of your home. For us, Emily gets her deepest sleep during the early morning hours. And thankfully, I'm somewhat of a functioning human being in the mornings. So it made sense for me, after the baby was well-fed but squirrelly, to get up before dawn and help him sleep through the rest of the night, giving Emily some much-needed REM. For others, maybe it's cooking or making sure the house is in some kind of order. Most of all, just be there and ready to answer the call when needed. You never know, it may be the perfect time to watch an incredibly depressing movie that your wife will never sit through again because it gave her nightmares. Just make sure the baby is asleep first. He's definitely not ready for *There Will Be Blood*.

CHAPTER 9

❀❀❀❀

A Crunchy Home Requires Sunshine

You know what's probably not going to happen when you're sitting on your couch vegging out to reruns of *Friends*? Snake bites. Tick bites. Mosquito bites. Why do so many things in nature want to bite you? If it's not looking to bite you, maybe it wants to sting you, give you a rash, poison you, or even poop on you! I get it, it's scary out there . . . it's called "the wild" so, yeah, things can get pretty *wild*.

When my husband and I were camp hosts at Prairie Creek Redwoods State Park in California, the park ranger told us that a few years prior, an older couple was attacked by a mountain lion on one of the trails. It took ahold of the husband's head, and he shouted for his wife to grab the ballpoint pen out of his pocket and stab it in the eyes. She tried to do what he instructed, but the pen didn't work, so instead, the couple fought off the mountain lion with a branch. Amazingly, the man survived.

I wanted to reply, "Thank you so much for that orientation. If you'd be willing to show me where the washing machine is, I have a little laundry to do before we pack up our RV and get the heck out of here." But the park ranger assured us attacks were extremely rare. We were more likely to drown in our bathtub or get struck by lightning than to be attacked by mountain lions. She just wanted us to be aware that they were out there.

Well, I don't know about you, but I want to be more than aware of mountain lions. What's the scout motto? "Be prepared!" So, according to the Mountain Lion Foundation (don't you love how there's a foundation for everything?), here's what you should do if you encounter a mountain lion: "Maintain eye contact. Stand tall. Look bigger by opening your coat or raising your arms. Slowly wave your arms and speak firmly. Throw items at the lion if necessary."[1] Now that you're prepared for mountain lion encounters, don't you feel inspired to get outside? I feel it—you're going to take on the thousand-hours-outside challenge starting tomorrow, aren't you? Okay, maybe a thousand hours is a lofty goal, especially if you hate being outside. But you know what else likely won't happen when you're sitting on your couch, vegging out to reruns of *Friends*? You won't increase your physical, mental, and emotional well-being.[2] These are all real, measurable, studied benefits of getting outdoors.

It's not a new idea that getting outside makes you feel happier and healthier. Throughout historical literature, it's well documented that when people were ill or having a mental health crisis, they were sent to the countryside for fresh air and sunshine. These people didn't need to sit down and read scientific studies to see the positive effect nature can have on us.

A difference between now and the days of yore is that we have something pulling us in, keeping us inside. We have screens. Many experts believe that certain kinds of screen time trigger such a large dopamine release in our brain's reward pathway that it is comparable to the addictive dopamine high achieved through the use of heroin or meth.[3] Screens are altering the way our brains work. That's some heavy knowledge, especially when we see it through the lens of raising children. No well-meaning parent, grandparent, or caregiver wants to negatively impact their child, but that's what is happening when we give kids free rein of unregulated screen time. The AAP recommends no more than two hours per day of screen time for kids ages six through seventeen. But the CDC reports that children in that age range are spending an average of seven and a half hours per day in front of a screen for entertainment, not including other educational screentime.[4]

Kids spending time in front of screens has become so normalized that you almost can't go anywhere without seeing a kid using their own device. Yet scientific studies are showing time and time again that screen time is bad for brain development. A study published in *JAMA Pediatrics* found that children ages three to five who were exposed to screens for more than the recommended one hour per day had less development of the brain's white matter.[5] This is the part of the brain where the development of language, literacy, and cognitive skills happens, and screen time is inhibiting its growth. Dr. Hutton, pediatric specialist and author of the brain matter study, said, "It's not that the screen time damaged the white matter. . . . Perhaps screen time got in the way of other experiences that could have helped the children reinforce these brain networks more strongly."[6]

I wonder what those experiences could possibly be? Oh yeah, *playing*! Even better, playing outside! You don't have to be a kid to play outside. Children and adults who spend more time outside are physically healthier than those who don't. As pediatricians Danette Glassy and Pooja Tandon explain, "More outdoor time is linked with improved motor development and lower obesity rates and myopia (nearsightedness) risk. Safely getting some sun also helps make vitamin D that our bodies need to stay healthy and strong."[7] Higher levels of vitamins D are linked to lower rates of certain kinds of cancer, diabetes, cardiovascular disease, and dementia.[8]

Being outside isn't just good for your physical health, it's amazing for your emotional and mental well-being too. According to the American Psychological Association, "[Researchers] found that children who lived in neighborhoods with more green space had a reduced risk of many psychiatric disorders later in life, including depression, mood disorders, schizophrenia, eating disorders and substance use disorder. For those with the lowest levels of green space exposure during childhood, the risk of developing mental illness was 55% higher than for those who grew up with abundant green space."[9] If there were a pill you could take that promised tons of health benefits and protected you from tons of health risks, wouldn't you take it? Why should spending time in green space be any different? Parks are free and abundant.

South Korea has one of the highest average life expectancies in the world. Many factors contribute to this, but from living there, I know for sure that Koreans get outside. Whether it's hiking around a park or nonchalantly climbing a mountain, Koreans know how to embrace nature. They even have calisthenics workout parks at the top of mountain trails. I've never felt like more of a wimp than when I was winded from climbing a mountain and I looked over to see an eighty-year-old marching away on a mountaintop elliptical.

Common Trends among Countries with the
Highest Life Expectancy

1. Keep faith at the forefront.

   Those who believe in a higher power believe they aren't in control of everything. They find peace in knowing they don't have to carry the weight of the world on their shoulders and can let go of daily stressors with the belief that everything is part of a greater plan. Less chronic stress often contributes to a longer life.

2. Prioritize family.

   Put family first. People in these countries often live near parents and grandparents to maintain a support system. They pour into their children and work hard to keep a connection with them.

3. Find community.

   A sense of belonging is a basic human need. Everyone wants to feel accepted and a part of something. This is often one benefit of being near

family or joining a church or a club. It feels good
to be wanted and also to contribute to something
outside yourself.

4. Keep moving.

People in these countries walk, work, and
stay active instead of vegging out on the couch.
Movement helps maintain strength, flexibility, and
fitness, which all contribute to longevity.

5. Get rid of stress.

This goes hand in hand with all the other points.
Stress leads to myriad illnesses. Find a healthy way
to deal with stress through getting outside, praying,
meditating, joining a club, or exercising. Find what
fills your cup and do it. Natural stress relief is usually
cheaper and more effective than therapy.

6. Eat less.

The healthiest countries have a lower BMI than
average. Their focus on healthy, nutrient-dense
foods helps them maintain a healthy weight, which
contributes to living longer.

7. Eat a lot of plants.

Lots of people in these countries have kitchen
gardens and eat produce they grow themselves.
They focus on eating lots of vegetables and whole
grains, essentially following the Mediterranean diet,
which has been recognized as one of the healthiest
diets in the world for half a century.

I host a Forest Friends group in my area where a group of moms meet together once per week to explore the outdoors and encourage our kids to marvel at the wonders of nature. I usually try to plan some sort of activity, and at a recent meetup, I drew a hopscotch board, had a jump rope available for jumping, and brought enough kites for everyone to fly. Everyone's demeanor lit up at the prospect of so many old-fashioned activities. Even my six-year-old noticed and proclaimed, "Look, Mom! Everyone is so happy!"

Before the dawn of twenty-four-hour television, children were forced to be creative because they didn't have access to constant entertainment at the push of a button. Without having something catered to them at every moment, they were forced to come up with entertainment on their own. One of the beautiful things about allowing our children to be bored is that it allows them to master creativity. Kids don't need kites and jump ropes or planning and materials to play outside; nature provides endless opportunities for fun.

My husband's grandmother has told me stories of when she was a girl growing up in the mountains of North Carolina. She and her friends found entertainment in flowers, sticks, leaves, and simple homemade toys. They would sail little pretend fairies down the creek on the broad leaves of irises. They would make an impromptu mud kitchen out of an old bowl, filling it with yard scraps and making mud pies. They could turn a group of bushes into a grand playhouse where they would play for hours. I asked her what one of her favorite memories was, and she said every Easter all the kids in her mill village were given permission to ditch their shoes, and they would go bare-foot until Labor Day.

Simple Childhood Games

- Kick the can
- Flashlight tag
- Duck, duck, goose
- Hide-and-seek
- Four square
- Monkey in the middle (Okay, as a short person I hated this game.)
- Red Rover (I suppose this one was banned from the schoolyard for a reason.)

Bring back these games by getting outside and playing them with your kids.

Being barefoot outside (also known as grounding) has been shown in scientific studies to have numerous benefits,[10] including:

- Improved sleep and cortisol rhythm
- Reduced pain
- Reduced stress
- Healthier nervous system
- Increased heart rate variability

- Faster healing
- Reduced risk of cardiovascular and cerebrovascular disease

It's no wonder my husband's grandmother is in her mid-nineties and living on her own. Playing outside, especially when barefoot, increases the microbial diversity that is a key component in immunity, gut health, and long-term health. One teaspoon of soil has up to a billion different diverse bacteria. Globally, people are oversanitizing their indoor environments with cleaners that offer to kill 99 percent of bacteria; then those same people are spending the majority of time inside these nearly sterile environments, which negatively impacts their microbial diversity. That is easily remedied by getting outside.

Being outside also builds resilience. I have seen this first-hand time and time again with my children. While Kentucky generally has very mild winters, last year each Forest Friends meetup for the first three or four months of the year seemed to hold some sort of curse for being the coldest or rainiest day of the week each and every week. The weather could be sunny with a high of seventy-five Monday through Wednesday, and for some reason by Friday, it would be below freezing. Nevertheless, we bundled up and got out there. Some weeks families showed up only to flee back to their vehicles after realizing how cold it really was. My family and another family continued to try our best to tough it out. If we were too cold, we found movement helped us warm up. Sometimes it felt like a healthy competition—if they could make it, so could we.

With the right clothing, being out in the cold wasn't terribly uncomfortable. It forced us to experience new sensations that showed us how much more outdoor time we are capable of.

Developing grit isn't a bad thing. We have become too conditioned with cushy lives and accessible comfort. When you start doing something outside the norm, you realize that normal doesn't always equal right. Just because something is difficult or a challenge doesn't mean it's bad or that it should be avoided.

Have you ever decided to leave your phone in the car when you go somewhere? I encourage you to give it a try. Look around and see how many people are looking down at their screens wherever they go. We have become so reliant on constant input and entertainment from a little box with lights in it that we are missing everything that really matters. I saw a video by Carly Rose, creator of rewildcarlyrose on Instagram, that really resonated with me. She said "Humans are not meant to wake up in a box and stare at boxes, eat out of boxes, drive to work to work in a box, while staring at boxes, going home to our boxes to stare at more boxes all day. This is not normal and humans are not meant to live like this."[11] All these boxes are causing us to miss the breathtaking displays that God has given us through nature to mark the passage of time. If you want to start thinking outside the box, step outside and wonder at the intricacies of nature.

As a child, I spent way too much time in front of the television and wasn't aware of the magic that awaited outside. As an adult, I am learning so many fascinating things that I never would've thought to try to figure out if I hadn't sparked my curiosity by going outside and taking a closer look. With all the benefits, it should be easy to make the choice to get out there, but people aren't. That's why the addiction to screens seems to be such an important piece to the puzzle of why people don't spend more time outside.

It's up to you to make the change for yourself and your family. If disconnecting from screens and getting outside more takes hiding the television in the basement, do it! Let's make hanging art on the wall more common than hanging televisions. Let's normalize holding books instead of holding phones. Be that crazy person who gets excited about all the things nature has to offer. When our Forest Friends group goes on a walk, I'm all, "Oh! Look guys! Look at all this lichen. How exciting!" and "Whoa! Look at that hole in that tree. Do you think something lives in there?" To me, exploring nature feels like the best Easter egg hunt, except it's never-ending and doesn't include Laffy Taffy—thank goodness.

This is one reason thousands of families have decided to take on the thousand-hours-outside challenge. According to Ginny Yurich, creator of the challenge, "The entire point of 1000 Hours Outside is to attempt to match nature time with screen time. If kids can consume media through screens 1200 hours a year on average then the time is there and at least some of it can and should be shifted towards a more productive and healthy outcome."[12] There is no denying that our children are spending too much time on devices. No matter your age, skin color, socioeconomic background, or other demographics, the truth is, less screen time and more green time will make you a happier, healthier person.

My husband and I went to an event where children's programming was offered. We are pretty picky (okay, really very picky) about who can keep our kids, but we knew the teacher of the kids' program, and strenuous efforts were put into vetting who could even come into the children's area. We had gone to this event before, there was a whole check-in process, and it felt safe. When we returned after an hour of the seminar to check on our boys, we found our children sitting in a chair with a boy who had a tablet in his lap. I was pretty upset. We are not only very picky about the types of media our children consume but also conscious about limiting it to appropriate times. We ended up not staying for the rest of the seminar because I didn't like what I saw in that moment. Here were three kids sitting in a chair staring down, with terrible posture, at something fake when there was a whole room of real toys and real opportunities for development and connection they were ignoring. I imagine this is the reality for many children and adults: people spending their lives consuming content instead of making memories, letting their lives pass them by.

I have come to realize that seeking out new interests and engaging in challenging pursuits not only invigorates my intellect but also provides a profound sense of contentment. Can you honestly recall an instance when spending countless hours in front of a television screen left you feeling truly gratified? Admittedly, I am a sucker for the exhilaration that accompanies immersing myself in an enthralling show or movie. But does this ritual have to be repeated night after night? Of course, there's an even worse ritual: the prolonged evenings devoted to mindlessly scrolling on the phone. You probably don't even get a good story out of that, and you certainly don't feel like you accomplished anything when you finally set down the phone far past the time to go to bed.

Early on in my relationship with Jason, we watched a lot of television. I like to think that marathons of *Seinfeld*, *Friends*, *Frasier*, *The Office*, and *Parks and Recreation* ultimately served us well since we both now write and film comedy for a living, but I often consider how many hours those shows were and how I could have better spent my time. That's time I could have spent learning to make foods that would be incredibly healthy for us without breaking the bank or learning to make clothes that would last longer than the latest fashion from H&M. At the very least, I would be far better at knitting than I am. (I have a lot more trouble with knitting than I care to admit.)

Just for fun (and to my utter horror), I did the math on those five shows and discovered it took up about five hundred hours of my life. If we were generous and said we watched two hours of television per night, then that's 250 evenings of sitting in front of a television! And that's not even counting regular content consumption. What could I have mastered in half a year? I hate the reality of math sometimes. Especially since I know these aren't the only shows I have binge-watched.

Time is a precious commodity, yet it is so easy to squander. No, it is not wrong to involve yourself with entertainment, especially when enjoying those things with someone you love. But again, life is about balance, and our society's standard consumption is not at all in balance. Having a life that is in balance requires making healthy choices every single day. So get outside with your family. See what discoveries nature has to offer. Use your imagination and enjoy the real world around you. I don't think you'll regret it.

What's your favorite outdoor activity?

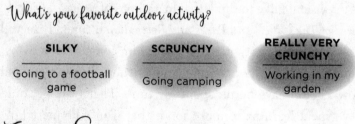

SILKY

Going to a football game

SCRUNCHY

Going camping

REALLY VERY CRUNCHY

Working in my garden

Jason Says ◀◀◀◀

Emily and I get our two boys outside as much as possible, and this has invoked a love for critters in both of them. Now, don't get me wrong, I love animals, but that doesn't mean I want them in my house. Or brought to me. Or asked to hold them. This was especially true when our three-year-old walked up to the house one day carrying a snake by its tail. I was inside editing a video and I heard him yelling, "Dada, oh Dada!" in the tone of, "I've got your worst fear right here in my hands. You want to see it?"

I love camping. I love hiking. I love seeing animals in the wild. I *hate* snakes. It has been a fear of mine since I can remember. No, I don't have trauma associated with snakes. I have never been bitten. I just can't stand them. Give me spiders. Give me any four-legged animal with sharp claws and teeth. But keep the snakes away.

Here's the problem. As the dad, I won't impose that same

terror on my three-year-old, who, when I opened the door, had the biggest smile on his face as he held the slithering reptile.

It was a green snake. Harmless, I knew, but it was still as snake.

"Want to hold it?" he asked.

I took a deep breath, smiled, and told myself (silently) that I could do this. I reached out and held it, mustering the strength not to chuck it across the yard.

I can only imagine what he's going to bring to the front door when he's ten.

SECTION 4

Crunchy Every Day

CHAPTER 10

Beauty Is in the Eye of the Beholder

I bet you know exactly what I'm talking about when I say gas station carnations. You know, the flowers you find at the counter at service stations that have been dyed an array of neon colors. When you see them, you think, "There's no way that's natural." Even if the colors are fun and punchy, you're left wondering why someone felt the need to try to improve upon the natural beauty of a fluffy, ruffly, dainty flower. The hot-pink and neon-blue blooms have cheapened carnations to being a "vase filler," a less desirable blossom, forever marred by the aesthetic found only inside the walls of a gas station. Why couldn't we leave it as it was?

I'm left asking myself the same question about the standards of beauty set for women. Why is society constantly trying to improve on and alter the natural form of our bodies and our faces? Gone are the days when Pond's Cold Cream

143

was the secret to beautiful skin (not that I'd recommend it, with some of the current ingredients). Now more and more women are opting for more extreme measures to mark new standards of beauty. And these aren't only women in their thirties and forties clinging to the last remnants of youth. Teenagers, people who are barely beyond childhood, are also concerned with signs of aging and are going so far as to get Botox and fillers. What has happened?

Augmented reality filters and the ever-growing obsession with social media exacerbate the problem. Society has set the bar so high that even the "most beautiful" people get photoshopped. I think the first step to breaking the cycle of physical dissatisfaction is recognizing that beauty is found in diversity. We shouldn't all want to look the same. We are not mass produced. That would be weird and creepy, and saying it feels like the perfect start to a post-apocalyptic novel. We are all uniquely, individually crafted inside our mothers' wombs, like beautiful works of art. Can you even look at a baby without admiring how precious they are? Their tiny little fingers and toes and nose—all so wonderfully made. Each person around you was a baby once; can't we look at them (and ourselves) with the same wonder and admiration? I mean, don't go around saying "Hey, baby!" to everyone you meet, but notice how amazing the human body is and how each body was created differently and has grown differently.

Notice lines on faces that signify sorrows and joys, physical markings of someone's story. A bit of a rounded belly that symbolizes a stretched womb and life brought forth. Tired eyes, a sign of parenting through the night. Sagging breasts, a sign of a baby nourished, loved, and connected to its mother. The opportunity to age is a gift.

It took me some time to accept this. I am one of the lucky ones who started getting forehead wrinkles in her twenties. Maybe I wasn't properly nourishing myself, maybe I was dehydrated too often, or maybe I'm an extremely demonstrative person who uses her facial expressions as a main source of communication. Maybe it was a combination of all of those factors plus a genetic disposition to wrinkles, but whatever it was, I got 'em, and I have had to fully embrace that they are a part of who I am. Sure, I wear wrinkle tape at night to keep my face from squishing because no matter how much I try to train myself, I can't sleep on my back all night long. Though now I'm starting to rethink that since I am preaching about being thankful for joys and sorrows and a life well lived; shouldn't I be thankful for a good night's sleep? I suppose you have to draw your line somewhere. Mine is with my quickly deepening elevens.

Acceptance of societal imperfections doesn't mean you shouldn't take care of yourself. It's not wrong to try to look and feel beautiful, but here's my unpopular opinion: if it consumes your thoughts and you can't accept who you are without getting injections of a known neurotoxin[1] (Botox) or implanting something that is known to be linked to an increased risk of lymphoma, autoimmune illnesses, joint pain, myopathy, brain fog, and more (breast implants are simply a bad idea), then you might need to do some inward work to discover what defines you. I love this quote by Robin Givhan, a writer for the *Washington Post*, who hit the nail on the head when she wrote, "The greater the distance between one's natural attributes and the beauty ideal, the greater the risk in reshaping, retraining and redesigning oneself."[2] Is it worth all the risk?

Procedures aren't the only beauty-industry offerings that carry risks; it's sometimes frightening to think of all the ingredients that are allowed to make their way into products. For the longest time makeup brands used Red Dye No. 3 in products, until it was found to cause cancer in lab rats, so it was banned from the beauty industry. For the record, it is still found in more than 2,900 foods, including many candies, strawberry-flavored milk, and cherries found in kids' fruit cups. According to the Environmental Working Group (EWG), "Since 2009, 595 cosmetics manufacturers have reported using 88 chemicals, in more than 73,000 products, that have been linked to cancer, birth defects or reproductive harm."[3] Even chemicals in makeup that are deemed "safe" absorb into your pores and enter your bloodstream. That's not very pretty, which is why I am careful about what I put on my skin.

Remember being in high school and getting ready to go to the mall or a dance or a game and doing the walk-through perfume application? My friends and I would create a cloud of fragrance with approximately twelve squirts of the latest and greatest body mist and then walk through it, likely breathing it in as we did so. We each took turns with the misting, so we are talking more like forty-eight pumps of synthetic chemicals into the air on any given day. I get a headache thinking about it now. I looked up the ingredient list of my favorite body mist from back in the day, and it contained some of the chemicals from that list of eighty-eight. I'm not even going to try to find the ingredients from the mega-makeup set my parents bought me from Claire's when I was in the sixth grade. It had every-thing: 150 eye shadows, 22 lipstick shades, 5 lip gloss shades, 7 shimmer eye shadows, 5 different bronzers. I remember pulling out the makeup map that listed what each tiny little product was—it was even more exciting than looking at that paper that comes in a box of assorted chocolates so you know what each flavor is. I remember seeing a booklet full of ingre-dients and tossing that to the side, but I can imagine the horror that my future self would've felt seeing ingredients containing ethanolamines, phthalates, formaldehyde, and parabens. The horror likely would've matched the sheer ecstatic joy I felt when opening that pink faux patent leather Caboodle knock-off. At least our bodies were created to be efficient at detoxing when the proper steps are taken.

My first foray into "clean" beauty was swapping from a spray can of dry shampoo to organic cocoa powder mixed with organic arrowroot powder. Notice *clean* is in quotations because this swap can certainly get a little messy. You can use these ingredients on their own or together, depending on the color of your hair and how much you want to smell like choco-late. Who wouldn't want to smell like chocolate? It's probably the most beloved food on the planet. Plus, you'll only smell like chocolate when you're rinsing your hair in the shower. But, considering that a recent study found that 70 percent of dry shampoos tested contained high levels of the cancer-causing ingredient benzene,[4] I felt good about my chocolaty swap.

The rise in awareness of the toxicity of makeup has made clean, holistic beauty products far more accessible. You can even find cleaner options at major retailers like Walmart,

Target, and Ulta Beauty. My favorite sources for searching nontoxic beauty products are www.thefiltery.com and www.ewg.org. Both of these websites have tons of free information about what to avoid and why. Obviously, as with every decision, it's up to you to read labels and make informed choices. Only you can decide what's best for your family.

Really Very Crunchy Makeup Swaps
That Might Make You Hungry

1. Potatoes for depuffing under eyes
   Here's how: The high levels of starch in potatoes plus the presence of vitamin C make them ideal for decreasing inflammation and puffiness. Just cut thin slices of a potato and stick them in the freezer for a few minutes, then place the cold slices on your eyes until they warm up.
2. Cocoa powder for eyeliner
   Here's how: In a small bowl mix a spoonful of cocoa powder with a few drops of water or liquid coconut oil to create a thick paste. Use an ultrafine eyeliner brush to apply the paste along the top of your upper lash line.
3. Spirulina for a funky eyeshadow
   Here's how: Mix a small amount of spirulina powder with a few drops of water and apply the blend using a clean fingertip or eyeshadow sponge.

4. Nutmeg for a bronzer

   Here's how: Mix 1 teaspoon of nutmeg with 2 teaspoons of arrowroot powder and apply the powder
   using a blush brush. You can adjust the color by adding
   a teaspoon of cinnamon or turmeric to the powder.
5. Berries for a lip stain

   Here's how: Use fresh or thawed-from-frozen
   blackberries or raspberries to rub on your lips to add
   stain. Be mindful in application as berries can stain
   your clothes.

As with food, the best choice for beauty products often lies with simplicity. This is one reason I like to support small businesses when choosing personal care products. These family-run businesses don't have access to or the desire to add to their products all the lab-made chemicals often found in mass-produced cosmetics. One of my favorite companies, Bigwoods Organics, runs a small organic farm in the woods of New Hampshire. The plants and flowers in their products are all wild harvested from their land or grown in their gardens. The milk and eggs found in their soaps and ovum oil come from their pasture-raised goats and chickens. It sounds so idyllic and romantic that I get to be one degree away from the products I use on my skin. Many small family operations like this are out there, so find one you love and want to support. It's a gratifying feeling to know you're directly supporting someone's livelihood and also purchasing something that's good and nourishing for your body.

You can even take matters into your own hands and make your own products. Doing so doesn't require you to have a farm, since many of the ingredients needed to make your own cosmetics can be found at the grocery store. Some foods that are beauty powerhouses include avocado for face masks, apple cider vinegar for a hair rinse, and milk for moisturizing and clearing away dead skin cells. Support a local meat farmer and buy chicken to make homemade jiggly bone broth, a superb source of collagen. If you want to be really very crunchy, find someone with an elderberry bush and ask if you can forage their berries. Then you can not only make one of the best natural immune-boosting tonics, elderberry syrup, but also use the berries for lipstick or cheek stain (if they say yes, that is).

Confessions of a Crunchy Mom

Coconut oil isn't a cure-all. I know that was a big thing for a while. Back when Facebook was more than just perfectly tailored ads, people fighting over whatever the latest national disaster is, and boomers sharing all the recipes, I remember many viral posts about how coconut oil could transform your life. In the words of Maury, "That was a lie," but organic coconut oil is an MVP when it comes to natural beauty hacks. You can use it as a moisturizer, deodorant, breath freshener via oil pulling, hair mask, natural lube, and shaving cream, plus it makes the very best makeup remover.

This chapter could probably be an entire book of recipes and natural cosmetic beauty hacks, but there is so much more to beauty than makeup and skincare products. I know we've all heard this sentiment, but I think few of us have really listened: what makes someone truly beautiful isn't their high cheekbones, their perfect eyebrows, or their physique. It's what's on the inside reflected outward that makes someone beautiful. You can't choose your physical flaws, but you can choose your personality strengths. Even if you have thin lips or crooked teeth, you can be kind. If you have a forehead full of wrinkles like mine, you can still be generous. You don't need perfect hair to be gentle or patient. Anyone can be honest, reliable, trustworthy, and helpful. Anyone can choose to be loving to those around them. Choosing the path of integrity isn't always easy, but pain is beauty, right? You don't have to be the prettiest person in a room, and knowing that takes a lot of pressure off. You can take the energy and finances from the obsessive pursuit of beauty (we all know it's not cheap) and funnel these resources into something much worthier.

What do you need to complete your outfit?

SILKY	SCRUNCHY	REALLY VERY CRUNCHY
Perfume	My Birkenstock sandals	Natural fibers and lime juice deodorant

Jason Says ——————————— ‹‹‹‹-

"We can't post this video! I look awful! The light is hitting my face all wrong."

This was Emily while I was editing one of our early videos for Really Very Crunchy—the one where Emily goes over to "Zane's mom's" house. That was back when we filmed with a phone and we were posting a video every day. I looked at the screen and shook my head.

"You look great. What are you talking about?"

I didn't see what she saw. When she said the angle made her look like Emperor Palpatine from Star Wars, I was incredulous. I finally convinced her to post the video since we didn't have anything else, but she hated that video so much.

Later, when I started being on screen, in one of the shots I was in the same place as she was in that early video. And I didn't like the angle when I was editing. I now saw what she didn't like because I saw it on myself. That earlier video had become known to us as the Zane's mom incident. So now, even to this day, if the light in our living room is questionable during filming, Emily will occasionally ask, "Do I look like Zane's mom?"

It's funny to think that how we look to ourselves doesn't necessarily reflect how we look to others.

CHAPTER 11

Don't "Waste" Your Life

Remember the song "Barbie Girl"? Who knew millennials would take the claim of a fantastic life wrapped in plastic to heart and cling to them, adopting them as a guide for building their lives? Plastic is everywhere; we are living in plastic. We are wearing plastic: go check your clothes labels. If you aren't trying to avoid polyester, acrylic, and nylon, you'll notice your clothes contain them. We are eating and drinking plastic: single-use paper plates, coffee cups, and obviously water bottles leach plastic into our food. Not to mention storage containers and plastic wraps. We are cozying up in plastic: that super soft blanket you love is probably plastic. We are slathering ourselves in plastics as many cosmetics contain plastics. And when we are bored, we are chewing on plastic: one of the main ingredients in most chewing gum is polyvinyl acetate, a type of plastic that is also used to make plastic bags and water bottles. It's listed in the ingredients as "gum base." When I say everywhere, I mean everywhere.

Plastic isn't the only problem—paper takes the cake for being the most common item found in landfills. Then there are aluminum cans, disposable diapers, shoes, clothing, and more. Think about all the stuff you throw away. Even if you're going through the motions of recycling, most stuff sent to recycling isn't actually being recycled. A study done by Greenpeace revealed that less than 5 percent of plastic is being made into new things. Whether or not you believe in climate change, waste is irrefutably bad for our planet. The air we breathe is more polluted through production and disposal, our soil and water are being contaminated, the ocean is filling with trash—these are undeniable signs that our consumption has gotten out of hand.

I want to blame companies for all the waste, but some fault falls on the consumers. We have all become accustomed to fast, easy, and cheap. Can you blame someone for capitalizing on a situation? Somewhere along the way, we quit caring about quality and wanted the newest, the easiest, the latest and greatest—and more of it. On one hand, it is lovely that people aren't struggling as much as they once did. The necessity to "use it up, wear it out, make do, or do without" is no longer there because people have more resources, so they can go out and buy whatever they want whenever they want or need. However, this shift has caused a ridiculous amount of waste.

If everyone took some simple steps to reduce their waste,

even by a little, we could make a big difference. One of the easiest things you can do is start using cloth napkins and dishrags instead of paper napkins and paper towels. Not only are paper towels not recyclable, they also aren't sustainable. Even if they are from "sustainably sourced trees," there's nothing sustainable about cutting down trees to make a single-use product. Paper towels and napkins are produced using harsh chemicals such as chlorine and formaldehyde, both of which are known carcinogens. Not that I think the finished product likely contains enough of the chemicals to affect you (unless you're draining your bacon on it . . . then maybe), but the production of this product that is supposed to promote cleanliness is really dirty work.

This is the one time I will have a potty mouth in this book, but it needs to be said: most toilet paper is crap. Being a single-use paper product automatically makes it wasteful. And while some "eco-friendly" options are out there, they're not a great choice. Many of those contain BPA because the papers being recycled to create toilet paper are often thermal printed papers such as tickets, shipping labels, food cartons, and receipts. So toilet paper can contain BPA, plus chlorine and formaldehyde like paper towels, but many also contain:

- Petroleum-based mineral oils (being marketed as infused with lotion), which are known carcinogens
- Fragrances, which are bad news (remember chapter 2?)
- PFAS, which are badder than bad and can cause liver disease, kidney disease, cancer, and more health issues

All these things are enough to make you want to say, "Well, poop!" But healthier *and* more eco-friendly options are available. The very best option out there is a bidet. You can have a full-on bidet installed in your home, or you can go the more affordable route and get a toilet seat that has an attachment.

I feel a bit of PTSD recommending that, as I had a disgusting experience with a toilet seat bidet. First, I should inform you that Korea has the most diverse toileting options I have ever seen. You never knew what you would get when you used a public bathroom. Sometimes there were squatty potties, which were little more than a hole in the floor that you had to straddle and squat over. Sometimes they had full-size toilets with amazingly high-tech toilet seats that included built-in bidets with remotes as intricate as cable TV remotes (which I still cannot understand how to operate). I'm talking buttons for courtesy music so you don't broadcast what exactly is going on within your stall, seat warming, adjustable water pressure on the bidet, adjustable spray direction, and even a warm air dryer.

On one of our first outings there, I needed to make a pit stop in a restroom, and I was met with one such high-tech toilet. I had never seen anything like it and didn't even know what all the buttons could be. I did my business and turned around to flush. It was at that moment I wished I had learned Korean *before* immersing myself in the culture. Some of the buttons had Korean characters and some had pictures on them. One picture looked like water flowing, so I decided that was probably the flush button. I hit it and nothing happened, so I kept trying to discern what button it could possibly be. I heard a little *eeerrr* sound of something electronic moving, but I kept focusing on the remote. It was then that I noticed a little wand protruding from the toilet seat, and it dawned on me that my flowing-water button selection was for the bidet. I knew what was about to happen, and there was nothing I could do to stop it. I couldn't move out of the way fast enough; it was a very deer-in-the-headlights moment for me. I was sprayed in the face and chest by a multidirectional bum-washer wand. I wanted to give up and leave, but the evidence of my visit was still there staring at me, so I called out in desperation, "Does anyone in here speak English?"

A small child's voice answered. "Yes?"

"How do I flush?" I choked through laughter and the desire to cry.

"It's on the top," she said.

Of course it was. Right there, on top of the toilet, was a flush button. I had been so thrown by the remote that I hadn't even thought to look in the obvious place.

If you're not one for booty sprays and prefer to stick with TP, at least opt for 100 percent bamboo, which is the most sustainable plant to chop because of its quick growth that requires little water and no fertilizer and because it self-regenerates. This toilet paper doesn't require the same chemically dense processing as conventional TP, so it's better for you and the planet. But if you want to wear a crunchy badge, look into family cloth. It's not as creepy or gross as it sounds; it's usually cotton cloths that can be put in a container upon wiping, then washed and reused.

Let's Talk **Personal Care Products**

Cloth diapers have become commonplace, but you know you've reached the crunchy apex when you use reusable period-care products (like washable cotton pads or period underwear). In the United States alone, twelve billion pads and seven billion tampons are discarded each year,[1] which is a lot of waste when sustainable, healthier options are easily accessible. Tampons and pads are one more place companies expose innocent bystanders to harmful chemicals. They are often made with plastics, treated with petroleum-based oils, and made with cotton that has been sprayed with pesticides. With all that stuff getting absorbed by your most sensitive area.

Food and food containers make up a major part of our waste. Whether the food is packaged for sale at the store, delivered in fast-food packaging, or even carted inside the plastic bags you picked up to transport your groceries home, there is so, so much waste when it comes to food. Unless you're able to grow all your own food, you will have to buy some things that come in packages, but you can minimize your impact. The easiest switch you can make is using reusable grocery bags. I keep mine in my car so I always have them. After I put away my groceries, I run my bags out to my trunk so I don't forget them on my next shopping trip.

Something else you can do is stock up at the farmers market as much as you are able and even learn to can and preserve foods you buy there. You don't have to grow food to preserve it. Buy in bulk as much as possible. Make as many things from scratch as you can. If you can buy a ready-made product at the store, chances are you can make it. Things like sour cream, crackers, and mayonnaise can all be made at home without a lot of skill. Making your own versions saves money and packaging. When you don't have the option to make something, as often as you can, try to buy a version in glass packaging that you can then reuse for future food storage. I know there are concerns about lead in glass, so try to avoid buying things in colored glass.

Most importantly, set yourself up for success by making a meal plan and buying only the ingredients you need to make those meals (be sure to follow through with cooking). Learn to eat and enjoy leftovers. We eat our leftovers from the previous night's dinner for lunch every single day. This ensures we don't waste food and that we avoid buying more packages for the sake of convenient "lunch foods" like deli meats (which aren't good for you anyway).

Another big part of minimizing waste is shopping less. This is a radical idea these days, but you can choose to be satisfied with what you have. Do you *really* need a new phone case, or do you just want it? Does every vacation call for a new swimsuit, or could you use the same one several years in a row? Do you need new outfits for family pictures, or could you piece together something from clothes your family already has? What happened to borrowing? Be brave and ask your friend if you can borrow her dress, or ask your neighbor to borrow his ladder, or ask your mom to borrow her Bundt pan because how many Bundt cakes do you really plan to make? (Please be a responsible borrower, taking great care of the item and returning it promptly so we other borrowers can keep a good name for ourselves.)

A long time ago people didn't have the option to buy new—they had to mend their broken objects. A Japanese art called kintsugi is a gorgeous example of this. It is a method of repairing broken ceramics with gold, and it makes the piece even more beautiful and stronger than it was before it was broken. Kintsugi inspires me to be creative with mending, making the mend an art in itself. I embroider over holes in sweaters and repair ripped furniture with a patch of fun fabric. I've used colored thread to secure the leg on a chair that broke. In fixing things, you bring celebration and attention to imperfections, little quirks that make life beautiful.

If you must make a purchase, look for something second-hand before buying new. A friend of mine has a running joke that there are so many hangers at thrift stores that the world could stop producing them and there would be plenty to last forever. You can find almost anything on Facebook Marketplace or Craigslist. If you're weird about buying things from thrift stores or from people you don't know, ask people you do know if they are selling whatever you're in search of.

I never thought I'd be the type of person to promote buying secondhand. When I was in middle school, I attended a private school with all the wealthiest families in my city. I was there on scholarship, but I was expected to fit in and wear the same uniforms as the rest of the students. Our local thrift store had a section of hand-me-down uniforms for us scholarship kids. I remember flipping through, scouring the rack for uniforms that weren't embroidered with my peers' initials. Wearing faded clothing was one thing; wearing someone else's initials was a whole new level of embarrassing.

I remember being excited to find a skirt that looked barely worn and in the newest uniform style. I knew this was my chance to *finally* look normal. My dad pressed my uniform the next morning, as he always did, and I showed up to school beaming with pride over my new 'fit. That is, until the dean saw me. Our dean was a soul-crushing sort of guy. He was old school, from the days of Catholic school when nuns were accustomed to smacking the backs of hands with a ruler. He used hair oil to slick his combover to the right, which earned him the nickname Mr. Greaselle. He spotted my joy and knew right away I must be up to something. I tried to slink behind the Coke machine, but it was too late. He approached with a grin more wicked than the Grinch's and said, "Emily, how long is your uniform skirt supposed to be?"

I looked down. It was *close enough* to my knee. Everyone else got away with this length, but everyone else's parents kept the school afloat. I wanted to say, "Hey, listen, dude, I didn't alter this skirt. Blame Melissa or Natalie or Hunter or whoever this belonged to before me. I'm just trying to make it, man." I didn't. I held back sobs of embarrassment and said I'd call my mom and see if she could bring me a change of clothes. I also swore when I grew up, I'd get a job that made enough money so that I could buy all my clothes brand new at Aéropostale.

Sorry twelve-year-old Emily, you're still wearing hand-me-downs and thrift store finds, but you have more subscribers on YouTube than any of those classmates, so take solace in that. Oh wait, you don't know what YouTube is yet.

We are a generation of wasters, and we are raising our kids to be even worse. Even with my mindfulness on this subject, I hear my kids say things like, "It's okay, we can buy another one," when they don't take care of their things and break them. This is not the mindset I want them to have. I want to teach my kids to be good stewards of what they have, using everything to its fullest potential. As with any lessons we teach them, this has to be something we model ourselves. I especially see wastefulness around holidays and celebrations. Do we need to buy so much single-use junk to give as "cheap" gifts? They might be cheap for you, but what are the environmental implications? Set down the cellophane bags, put back the plastic tablecloths, stop buying so many balloons, and make do with what you have. Think about how your great-grandmother would've made holidays special. The best memories aren't made because of stuff; they are made because of moments of intention and connection.

What is your favorite Christmas tradition?

SILKY	SCRUNCHY	REALLY VERY CRUNCHY
Watching twenty-five Christmas movies in December	Driving through the park to look at the lights	Caroling in woolens while carrying beeswax candles

Jason Says ———————————— -«««-

Emily doesn't waste things. Have you seen the video we put out last year about the baskets? The one where baskets are stacked from floor to ceiling with all the ones she's collected over the years and I'm trying to stage an intervention? Some videos are made because we see the absurdity in our real lives. For this one, I pitched the idea to Emily, but she didn't think she had that many baskets. So while she was away, I went throughout the house, pulled out every basket from every shelf, corner, nook, and cranny until there was an entire wall of baskets. The moment she walked into the house, she knew it would be a good video.

Though in the video I stage an intervention, I never actually asked her to get rid of her baskets. They replace cheaper plastic storage bins that easily break. While some people may gather trash in plastic bags, a basket is just as easy to hold it, then dump it. I see the benefit. Plus, they look nicer. But man, we have a lot of baskets. There may be a fine line between "not wasting" and hoarding, but I'm not sure where it is.

CHAPTER 12

There Is a Natural Remedy for Almost Everything

Have you ever seen those ads for prescription drugs on TV? Why are there so many weird side effects? Sometimes the list doesn't sound so bad, but sometimes the side effects sound much worse than the symptom the drug proposes to treat. *Side effects may include dry mouth, hives, strong urges to gamble, bleeding out of every orifice, and sometimes even death.* I think I'll take my chances with seasonal allergies, thank you. Especially when there are basic low-risk options out there like consuming raw, local honey, taking colostrum, or removing certain triggers in your diet.

Our society has become so accustomed to "quick and easy" that we expect our health care and treatment options to align with that way of thinking as well. It doesn't help that the United States is one of only two countries in the world where pharmaceutical companies are allowed to market directly to consumers. We are inundated with advertising that lures us into popping pills to mask symptoms rather than dealing with the root cause. Think about the Larry the Cable Guy Prilosec commercials where he parades around eating deep-fried corn dogs, massive hamburgers, and fully loaded nachos. People were not meant to live on fair food alone. If those things give you heartburn, it's your body's way of saying, "Don't eat those things!" But it's okay because Larry the Cable Guy said it's fine to get on a daily pill that changes your body's chemistry so you'll never have to worry about it ever again.

In a time before twenty-four-hour CVS stores, people treated illness and ailments at home using generational wisdom that was passed down through the years. They didn't have to rush to the store for products if they were stung by a bee; they chewed up a piece of plantain leaf and stuck it on the sting for immediate relief. People grew gardens with herbs like mint for upset stomachs and chamomile for restlessness. People experienced all these things before there was the option of quick "fixes." Sure, there were pharmacies and apothecaries, but those often sold homemade salves, tinctures, and dried herbs and teas—not Prilosec or Tylenol.

I'm not proposing we go completely back to how things used to be—maternal mortality in childbirth used to be excessively high, and doctors would prescribe cocaine for something as simple as a toothache. Not everything our parents or grandparents did was the best choice either. My husband's grandmother said her son's pediatrician prescribed him pare-goric when he was teething. Paregoric is a tincture of opium, which explains why he rarely cried. But it's worth recognizing that sometimes our bodies are telling us to make changes in our habits or our environment, and instead of looking for a quick "cure," we can a take slower, more holistic approach to feeling better. Covering up or masking symptoms is not the same as healing.

One way I like to support my body is through the use of herbs. The boom in the popularity of essential oils primed people to feel empowered by plant medicine, but many are questioning the potency of essential oils as a safe choice. Some of those people have turned toward a simpler, whole-plant approach of herbal medicine. There are many great educational establishments out there that offer a fantastic introduction to herbalism, one of my favorites being theherbalacademy.com.

There is a place for community and shared experiences on social media, but it needs to be secondary. I'm part of a rather large crunchy mom Facebook group, and I have seen some pretty amazing interactions there, but having inter-actions with people whose eyeballs you're able to look into, face-to-face, is more important. A friend or family member you spend time with will likely have a more vested interest in the wellness of you and your family and therefore give more tailored advice. Find yourself a friend you can send rash pic-tures to—a reciprocal rash rendering relationship, if you will. But of course, keep in mind that Aunt Claudia can't point to a liver on a picture of the human body, so prioritize advice from practicing medical professionals.

I am one of the lucky ones who has generally very healthy kids. I take my kids to the doctor once a year to chart their growth and check their vision and hearing, but—aside from the time my son got a stick lodged in his throat—we have been able to care for most ailments on our own. Daily maintenance of their health through eating whole, nutrient-dense foods, avoiding too much sugar, and getting outside as often as possible to soak up that sunny vitamin D has served us well. There are consequences to eating overly processed foods and living a sedentary lifestyle. As parents, we have the responsibility to steward our resources and knowledge responsibly and try our best to set healthy habits for our kids. Does that mean they will never get sick? No. Often when they are sick, though, patience, hydration, and close monitoring are all that's needed to get them on their way to wellness. Obviously this will be different for different kids, but I encourage you to try not to be passive in your child's health care. It's your job to figure out what works for your kid and do your best to keep them healthy and safe.

There is a dark side of the crunchy world that is anti-doctor, but I think any levelheaded person who would call themselves crunchy knows there is a time and a place for natural and alternative wellness and the same is true for conventional medicine. Most crunchy moms aren't looking to purge doctors from their lives. Rather, they seek to find health-care providers they trust. I've had some experiences with allopathic medicine where I was treated like I was on an assembly line—doctors not viewing me as an individual person with unique needs but instead trying to meet a quota of how many people they could get through their door. Of course, that isn't the case for every doctor! The great news is, as a patient, you are the boss. If your provider isn't serving you in the way you feel is appropriate, you can find a new provider. I have an allopathic doctor friend who recommends her patients drink bone broth and take elderberry syrup before moving on to more aggressive treatments. I hate that some people feel everything has to be one extreme or another. A healthy life is found in balance and the use of quality information to drive your decision-making.

While I'm eager and excited to look for natural remedies, I'm counting on modern medicine to potentially save the life of my husband. Jason was diagnosed with polycystic kidney disease, a rare genetic kidney disease that may cause his kidneys to fail in the future. Though I want to do everything I can to help him stretch the life of his kidneys, there's no essential oil, tea, or tincture that will cure his kidney disease. There's very little research available on natural options that might help. Common sense tells us that a healthy, whole-food diet and exercise will go a long way in maintaining his general health, so that's our main plan while we wait and see what happens. But one day he may need a kidney transplant, and I am so thankful modern science has made that a possibility. Jason's dad had polycystic kidney disease as well, and Jason's mom was a perfect match for his dad. What a miraculous blessing! Truly a one-in-a-million chance that he would marry his perfect kidney match. Jason's dad used to joke that he kept her around for spare parts. I've told Jason he is welcome to one of mine if it works out that way. I can imagine how my wedding vows would have looked a little different if we had known he had this disease when we got married. "And I, Emily, promise you my left kidney to have and to hold . . ."

My mom, whose advice I generally trust, once told me that to avoid pain while breastfeeding, I needed to toughen my nips by roughening them up with a washcloth before I had my baby. This is something her mom, a successful breastfeeder of nine children, taught her. My mom exclusively breastfed all four of her children for more than a year each. I took her advice with my first son, and all I can say is ouch! That was a miserable few days after the roughening. If you've seen the show *The Office*, think of the episode where the whole office is going to do a charity run and Andy has sensitive nipples, so he does everything he can to avoid chafing but, in the end, runs with blood stains over his poor, chafed nipples. Yeah, that was me.

Once I had my son, I proudly proclaimed to the lactation consultant that I shouldn't have a problem with pain since I had done the job of toughening up, and she looked at me with horror in her eyes. Turns out, breastfeeding doesn't have to be painful—it's all about having the proper latch. A quick internet search reveals how this "toughening up" is a myth and how it can actually be harmful. I know now I should've done more to inform myself. Thankfully, it worked out for me, and I was able to have a pain-free breastfeeding journey.

Sure, there are general remedies that anyone can try with

very little risk, like elderberry syrup for cold-and-flu symptoms, homemade bone broth when you're coming down with something, or a plantain salve for poison ivy. But I steer clear of ordering supplements or products just because an influencer says it works. Not everyone is trying to mislead you, but I can tell you firsthand that companies are willing to pay big bucks to get their product out there through social media accounts. I had a popular oat milk brand offer to pay me $12,000 to make one TikTok video using their product as a swap for milk. I have used oat milk, and I like the taste. However, it's not actually a healthy alternative to milk, and this brand added canola oil to make it taste creamier. I couldn't in good conscience tell people to use that milk, even though it would have been an incredibly easy way to make a lot of money!

Be careful and thoughtful about who you take recommendations from when it comes to online personas. Make sure it's someone you've followed for a while and who you know isn't just using their platform to make money. Let me be clear: Influencers are not medical experts. And even if they have the credentials to be one, they are not your doctor. Take my account for example. I drop a lot of little health ideas here and there in my videos. I try to make informed decisions to care for my family, but please don't do something I mention in a video just because I'm doing it. Every individual needs to seek counsel from a qualified source and not some random person on Instagram or social media—that needs to be the very last place anyone would go for medical advice. Never take serious health advice from anyone other than a professional you trust.

Fire Cider

INGREDIENTS

1 onion, chopped

2 garlic heads, peeled and chopped

2 jalapeño or habanero peppers, chopped

1 chunk fresh ginger the size of your hand, grated*

1 fresh horseradish root, grated*

1 chunk fresh turmeric a few inches in size, grated*

1 whole lemon, chopped

1 bunch rosemary

1 cup raw, organic apple cider vinegar (more if needed
    to fill the jar)

1/4 cup raw, local honey

Add the onion, garlic, jalapeños, ginger, horseradish,
turmeric, lemon, and rosemary to a glass quart-size jar.
Pour the apple cider vinegar over the top to fill the jar.
Your sinuses should be clear after that task—whoa! Seal
the jar with a piece of parchment, keeping the vinegar
from touching the metal lid, or use a plastic lid if you
have one. Store it in a cool, dry place for a month, making sure to shake it daily. Strain the vinegar through a
cheesecloth or fine mesh sieve into a clean jar. Add the
honey and "enjoy" 1 to 2 tablespoons (up to three times

daily) when you need an immune boost. The vinegar
should keep for up to one year.

*You can substitute a tablespoon of powdered spice if you don't have access to fresh.

Small-Batch Elderberry Syrup

INGREDIENTS
1 cup fresh or frozen elderberries (half that if using dried)
4 cups filtered water
1 cinnamon stick
5 whole cloves
1 (3-inch) piece of ginger, grated
1 lemon or orange, sliced
½ cup raw, local honey

Add the elderberries, water, cinnamon stick, cloves,
ginger, and lemon or orange to a pot and bring the
mixture to a boil and then simmer until it is reduced
by half (about forty-five minutes). My family hates the
smell of this process, so brace yourself for complaints.
Remove the pot from the heat and allow the mixture to
cool to room temperature. Strain the liquid into a clean
jar and add the honey. The syrup keeps in the fridge for
two months. I like to freeze mine as small ice cubes and
thaw them when needed. Take a teaspoon up to three
times a day when you have a cold or flu. Elderberry
syrup can also be used for daily immune support.

Jiggly Golden Chicken Bone Broth

INGREDIENTS

Chicken carcass, cooked and stripped of its meat

Filtered water

Splash of apple cider vinegar

(Optional: carrots, onion, celery, rosemary)

Place the chicken carcass (bonus points if you include the skin, neck, and de-nailed feet) in a large stock pot. Cover the chicken with filtered water until the bones are about two inches below the waterline—too much water weakens your broth. Add in the apple cider vinegar plus optional vegetables and herbs. Bring the broth to a rolling boil, then reduce the heat to maintain a simmering boil until the liquid has reduced by half. Store in the fridge for three to four days or in the freezer for up to six months.

Knowledge is power. Information and education are means of empowerment for you to make whatever choices make sense for your family. It's important to remember that just because someone has different opinions than you doesn't mean their experience isn't valid, but you also don't have to do things the way they do them. There is no one-size-fits-all way of doing things. Even with herbal medicines and natural remedies, what works for one person won't always be what works for the next. That's why freedom and choice are such beautiful aspects of our lives.

How do you treat a cold or flu?

SILKY	SCRUNCHY	REALLY VERY CRUNCHY
DayQuil! Duh!	Drink a bunch of orange juice for the vitamin C	Up your beef liver intake and sit in the sun

Jason Says ———————————— -<<<<-

I am a natural skeptic of natural remedies. I come from a background of "God gave us brains to come up with these really great medicines, so what's wrong with them?" So when I hear about someone rubbing oregano oil on the bottom of their feet to ward off a virus, I still want to roll my eyes. (Please don't come at me oil people. I'm sure you've had great success.) That said, the last five years have really opened my eyes to just how much money medical and pharmaceutical companies stand to make. That's true for big natural remedy companies too. Everyone's looking to make a buck off your health woes.

As Emily wrote, I have polycystic kidney disease. So far it hasn't affected me too much, but my kidneys may fail in the next ten to twenty years. However, there is a drug out there that supposedly stops the progression of cysts on the kidneys, and you can live as though your kidneys are just fine. Except . . . the side effects.

Here's the deal. I could have perfectly healthy kidneys so long as I'm never five minutes away from a toilet (or a tree, but that doesn't really work on a neighborhood walk, does it?). The medicine they want me to use makes you so thirsty you can't ever quench your thirst. I truly hope I never have to go on that medicine, but if I do, I suppose it's better than kidney failure. There is a lot of good out there being done in the medical world. But there are a lot of bad players, so you have to take each situation as it comes. I just hope that by the time I need a new kidney, they are able to use pig kidneys. Preferably pastured pork, of course.

CHAPTER 13

Crunchy Self-Care

Have you ever seen Crater Lake? It's a gorgeous blue lake that was born out of the collapse of an ancient volcano in Oregon. Its intense beauty can be described as resplendent, bordering on otherworldly. It's like something seen on Instagram that has been so filtered you know it's not real, but this is very real.

Years ago I stood on the rim looking down through a screen while I took picture after picture trying to capture its beauty. The lens on a camera phone cannot do it justice. While I am grateful to have those pictures, when I close my eyes and think about my time there, all I see are those pictures. I'm not sure I can remember what the lake looks like through my own eyes. I wanted documentation, evidence I had been there, but it came at the cost of my actual memory of being there. I remember posting one such photo on my personal Instagram with the hashtag #nofilterneeded. Am I the only one who finds it interesting that we regurgitate trends in search of validation that what we are doing is cool, neat, desirable?

Travel can be a wonderful gift because it broadens your perspective on the world. You can feel like you have accomplished something by putting your body in another location. Talking to a well-traveled person often feels like talking to a vegan or a CrossFit addict; they can't help but bring it up! They'll let you know within minutes how experienced and worldly they are. This seems particularly true about people who have been to Bali. Am I jealous because I haven't been to Bali? Of course, but that's beside the point. I think what these people are seeking is not more stamps in their passport but the richness that comes from overcoming challenges and experiencing new things. They want a feeling of enlightenment and education. Unfortunately, we can't all travel the world over, so we look for other means of satisfying the innate desire to expand our minds. Modern conveniences, while great, have given us more time to feel restless, and in general, people seem less satisfied with their lives, always in search of ways to fill an emptiness that was once filled with the satisfaction of completing their daily rhythm.

Enter: self-care. You've heard the phrase "You can't pour from an empty cup," and that is so true. It is important to make sure you're nourishing your spirit, body, and mind, especially as a parent. However, there is a danger of slipping from filling up your cup so you can pour it out to others *to* making sure your cup is always full and never allowing anything to empty your cup because you're worth having a full cup. Somewhere along the way, we've gotten so used to the treat-yo-self mentality that treats are no longer treats—they have become common-place. Sadly, we have become a culture of pacification. We are becoming self-obsessed and practicing self-worship in the name of self-care. One way we have done this is through the excessive consumption of social media. Looking at beautiful pictures makes you feel creative and inspired, but in reality, you're left empty-handed unless you go forth and accomplish one of those Pinterest projects you've had pinned for eight years now. We are not meant to simply consume; we are meant to contribute. If you're looking to make healthier choices for yourself and your family, look past "self-care" and focus on picking up nourishing habits that will fill your cup in a way that allows you to pour out freely to others.

Put down your phone and plant some seeds. Gardening is an excellent way to expand your skills, feel a great sense of accomplishment, and overcome challenges. I haven't been to Bali, but I have experienced the feeling of planting zinnia seeds, watering them, and seeing the buds shoot up and then bloom into delicate, ethereal blossoms so perfect no artist has been able to capture the beauty I initiated and cultivated. There's no greater joy than watching my toddler pick tomatoes that we grew together and seeing him take a big bite out of one, juice running down his chin and onto his shirt. Whether it's flowers, food, or herbs, everyone can grow *something*.

Learn to bake bread. People have been baking bread for thousands of years. When you engage in a centuries-old practice, you can feel connected to the past. Bread making feels a bit like a ritual. It is repetitive and rhythmic. It's a fulfilling sensory experience, a practice of being in the present and enjoying it fully. This is the case for any type of baking or cooking. It's quite fulfilling to be able to take singular ingredients and transform them into nourishment and sustenance for your family.

Have you ever heard someone say the movie was better than the book? I have not! I refuse to believe it's possible because when you're reading, you get so wrapped up in the story it feels like you are part of it. Let's stop watching Netflix and twenty-four-hour "stories" on social media and start reading. Reading has long been documented as being good for you. Reading exercises your brain, increases your memory, and reduces stress (look at you go; if you're here, you're obviously on board). As my children get older, I want them to be able to avoid the lure of the screen. While I often find myself fighting a desire to check out of reality through scrolling, I know that the example I set for my children will make a lasting impression on them. I don't think parents would say they hope their kids grow up to be people who scroll. If I want them to read, I have to be a reader. This is probably strange advice coming from someone who makes a living through getting people to watch my videos online. I don't think all content consumption is evil, but I do think it's dangerous to allow it to become what you spend most of your time doing. I think it's a bad idea to replace reading and developing skills with scrolling. Set timers for yourself to manage your consumption. Choose to scroll during times when your kids are busy so it's not taking away from time that you could be present and connected with them. Don't waste time on consuming content that's not adding value to your life. Scroll responsibly.

Any part of the slow-living movement can contribute to a healthy take on self-care and nourishment. Find joy and accomplishment in creating your own cleaning supplies. Pamper yourself by making personal care products. Find beauty in daily tasks that bring joy. When you fill your time doing things that are meaningful to you, you're able to build a life that is interesting. Create beauty in rhythms and rituals. Make ordinary moments feel special. One of my favorite things in the world is fresh flowers on the dinner table. Picking flowers from my garden and mixing them with blooms I picked up at the farmers market feels indulgent. Putting down a fresh tablecloth and lighting a beeswax candle at meals reminds me how blessed I am. Create beauty around you and you won't feel the need to escape or as if you are losing yourself in the humdrum of everyday life. In this way of living, self-care becomes a by-product of living well.

There are some commonsense ways to make sure you're choosing good habits to nourish yourself. A friend of mine decided to join an exercise class. She wanted to make sure she was doing everything right and following the instructor as closely as possible. It just so happened this class was being live streamed for people who wanted to follow along from home, and my friend somehow ended up on camera. She was so focused on doing the moves perfectly that at one point the instructor lifted her arm to look at her watch while she was doing squats and my friend lifted her arm right along. She held her arm up the whole time and later realized what the instructor was doing and felt so embarrassed—she wasn't even wearing a watch. Caught on camera. Oh, what I would give to be one of the ones who got to see that. I have considered joining the gym to see if they catalog their live streams.

It takes guts to get out there and join a class! I am not consistent with working out, but I do try to live an active lifestyle. As a family we take walks after dinner each day, go for bike rides, and work in the garden, and I try to dedicate at least twenty minutes a day to hard-core playing with my boys. Of course they like games that require me to run and jump and move my body. By nature, we don't get out as much in the winter, and I can tell that each one of us suffers from the decrease in activity. Several scientific studies have shown that exercise reduces anxiety and depression and improves mood, self-esteem, and cognitive function.[1] No matter who you are, no matter the state of your mental health, exercise should be a top priority for taking care of yourself.

One of the best things you can do for yourself is get outside. I spent almost an entire chapter of this book touting the benefits of touching grass—it's that important. This is one reason I am such a big fan of the one-thousand-hours-outside challenge. While reaching a thousand hours spent outside over the course of the year is a fun goal for our family, it's not about getting to the thousand-hour mark; it's about pushing yourself to choose nature as much as possible. Eat lunch outside, eat dinner outside, play games in the yard instead of on the tablet—do whatever it takes to get out! As Ginny Yurich, the founder of the challenge, told me, "If you lose, you still win."

It's important to ask yourself where you are working against your body's natural tendencies. We weren't made to eat processed junk food and sit inside and stare at screens all the time. Just as nature has a rhythm of seasons, we should have a daily rhythm that supports our overall wellness so there is less of a feeling of needing to escape. It's natural and perfectly healthy to take some time to yourself when you can get it, but if that has become your obsession and goal, maybe you should evaluate what the deeper problem is. *Am I eating nourishing foods? Am I getting outside? Am I sleeping enough? Am I connecting with others?*

Being crunchy is about making the best decisions you can make with the resources available to you. That applies to a million little things—the air quality in your home, the food you buy for your family, the way you parent your children—and it's important to give yourself some space and grace to find balance.

What is your favorite way to treat yo self?

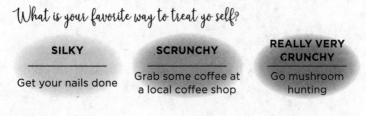

SILKY	SCRUNCHY	REALLY VERY CRUNCHY
Get your nails done	Grab some coffee at a local coffee shop	Go mushroom hunting

Jason Says ———————— -«««-

I really don't like working out. People keep telling me there's a point where you actually start to enjoy it, but I've never gotten there. The closest I've come is the runner's high you get after you've been running for several weeks, but those first few weeks are grueling. And is it just me who feels like they've been hit by a car after strength training for the first time in a while? Is that normal? I am more a fan of the hike-new-trails and climb-some-rocks workout routine, but those opportunities don't seem to come up often enough to be a routine.

I know the experts say that quality of life skyrockets when we work out, even just a little bit. Maybe some of you out there can try it and let me know if that's true.

CHAPTER 14

Beyond Crunchy

My husband and I have moved fifteen times in fourteen years of marriage. In most of the places we lived, we didn't have any family around—and let's face it, it's sometimes hard to make friends as an adult. I remember one time, when we were living in Wisconsin, a family that used to be friends with my parents (and had no association with me) heard that we were going to be alone on Thanksgiving, so they invited us to join them. They had a couple of other nonfamily members join, and I remember getting up to get some sweet potatoes and glancing back at the table. They were a motley crew of folks: loners, some with greasy hair, ill-fitted clothes, peculiar personalities. These were the people who had nowhere to go on Thanksgiving. These were the hard-to-love types, and I was lumped in with them.

My whole life I've had a friend or two who fell in the hard-to-love camp, sometimes because I was also in that camp and didn't have another choice of friend, and sometimes because I spotted them and knew they could use some companionship. When we moved back to my hometown (which is where we've been for the last seven years), I met one such person. She was single, in her seventies, and smelled strongly of patchouli. She was lonely and enjoyed spending time with me and my first son. Once, at a potluck, I saw her stir her dish of beans, then scrape the spoon with her teeth and stick it back in the pan. My stomach churned thinking of all the chia seed puddings and picnics we had shared together. If she was willing to lick the spoon at a potluck, she surely had licked all the spoons she used when cooking for us.

She passed away a couple of years ago, but when I miss her, sometimes I like to go back and read through our texts. One of the last things she sent me was "What a joy you are to me! A treasure that will shine forever!" I tear up with regret thinking of times I didn't want to hang out because she was a bit much. But I'm glad I did make time to be with her often, and oh, what I'd give for one last jar of her slimy chia seed pudding.

Research shows us that loneliness is on the rise and that a lack of human connection can be more harmful to health than obesity, smoking, or high blood pressure. Loneliness is linked to increased risk of cardiovascular disease and stroke. It's linked to elevated risk of early dementia and Alzheimer's. It should be no surprise there's a link between loneliness and depression, anxiety, and suicidal ideations. Overall, people who label themselves as lonely die younger and have more chronic diseases.

So many things polarize people these days. Whether it's your stance on food dye and fragrances or who should be elected and why, there are far too many opportunities for us to close others out and isolate ourselves in the name of seeking out a specific type of community. That's a recipe for loneliness on all sides. Instead, lean into investing in relationships with the people around you. Of course it's fun to meet someone who has common convictions and with whom you see eye to eye, but that's not what this life is about. We aren't supposed to be completely comfortable surrounded by agreeable people who support everything we do. People who see things differently than you can sometimes open your eyes to what really matters: showing love, being kind, having respect for others' life experiences that brought them where they are. What is the point of trying to live a healthier life if all it does is isolate you? Don't allow the desire to be toxin-free consume you so much it cuts you off from the rest of the world.

This has been a legitimate struggle for me. I haven't wanted to go out to eat with people or go to someone's house because of what and how they cook. What if they serve those store-bought cookies that are unnaturally soft and smothered in pastel icing with neon sprinkles? What if they offer my kids Capri Sun? What if they use nonstick pans and leave a plastic spoon in the hot pan? Or even worse, what if they cooked the meal in a worn slow cooker that's leaching lead, or what if they used a slow-cooker liner? *What if they serve us tap water?* As I type this, I can feel myself getting anxious just thinking about those things. I'm certainly prone to anxiety anyway, which is probably one of the reasons I choose the crunchy lifestyle: I learn new information and adjust my life accordingly, lest there be a consequence to pay. But what is so funny, so ironic, is that stress is far more damaging than any of the things I get anxious and stressed about. According to the American Psychological Association, stress affects all bodily systems, including musculoskeletal (muscle tension), respiratory (quickened and shallow breathing), cardiovascular (increased heart rate and blood pressure), and endocrine, gastrointestinal, nervous, and reproductive (stress hormone release). On top of that, new research shows stress is linked to tumor development and growth as well as the suppression of natural killer (NK) cells, which are "actively involved in preventing metastasis and destroying small metastases."[1] So, yeah, stress is awful for you. The key is to find a happy medium of making healthier choices without obsessing about it.

As someone who can get anxious just thinking about how awful anxiety is for you, I have a pretty good handle on how to control it. If I didn't, it would have gotten the better of me. In general, many people believe being outside is one of the greatest stress-relieving tactics out there. Nature is beautiful, rhythmic, and resilient. Seeing its resiliency gives me great comfort and hope. I also like to use self-talk to tell myself what I am doing to benefit my health: *I stay hydrated, I eat healthy food, I am mindful of my breathing, I go to an infrared sauna, I squish my toes in the mud.* Remind yourself of whatever it is you've done to make choices beneficial to your health. I try to be in tune with my body and recognize any signs of anxiety creeping in. For me, my forehead feels tight, my throat feels like someone is grabbing it, my core gets a burning sensation, and I'm not able to shift my thoughts away from whatever is bothering me. During those moments, I take a big, deep breath and pray, "Holy God, I surrender this worry to you. Your will be done over this." I cannot control every aspect of this life, so I have to stop trying. I can only make educated decisions. I then look at my situation and ask, "What is true right now, in this very moment?" The truth is my children are healthy, I am healthy, and we are safe. You can only do what you can do, and that's enough.

Another way I fight stress is actively choosing joy. There are obvious health benefits to choosing joy, focusing on the blessings we have been given, and having a glad heart. In life we are going to experience pain, trauma, and difficulty—those are natural parts of living. Everyone will experience suffering to some degree, but we shouldn't allow ourselves to stay there. According to the Mayo Clinic, "[Gratitude] can improve sleep, mood and immunity. Gratitude can decrease depression, anxiety, difficulties with chronic pain and risk of disease."[2] Put in the simplest terms, anxiety and worry are the worst things you can do for your health. Choosing joy and gratitude and connecting with others are some of the best things you can do for your health. Don't allow an attitude of negativity, anxiety, or superiority become more toxic than the toxins you are trying to remove from your life.

What is the best form of stress relief?

SILKY	SCRUNCHY	REALLY VERY CRUNCHY
A bath bomb!	Diffusing lavender essential oil	EFT Tapping and breath work

Jason Says —————————— -««-

"Oh my gosh, can I get a picture with you?"

That's what we often hear when Emily and I are in public and someone recognizes us. They then promptly put an arm around Emily and hand me their phone to take the picture. (When I get asked to be in a picture, people often say they think their husbands would think it's hilarious.) Neither Emily nor I ever thought the impact of Really Very Crunchy would be this big. This whole thing started because we thought it would be funny to make videos about Emily's crazy crunchiness. As Really Very Crunchy has grown and grown, we have met people from all walks of life saying how much they love the content, how much they identify with Emily, or how they now understand where some of their friends or loved ones are coming from. We've heard moms say they struggled to connect with their daughters until they had the mutual discovery of our videos. We've had many, many people reach out asking what they can do to be "really very crunchy." I just want to say, we love every bit of it. It's such an encouragement to meet you out in the real world and take pictures and put faces to the names we see online. Each and every one of you has been a blessing to us, and we couldn't be more grateful.

Conclusion

I don't know what you may have expected when you picked up this book. Maybe you sought the company of the judgy Emily, whose piercing gaze would cast a shadow of disapproval upon your iced caramel latte due to its unholy blend of homogenized milk and nonorganic, glyphosate-ridden coffee.

Perhaps you were hoping for a tough kick in the backside to get you started on the journey you should have started a long time ago because (obviously) the world is falling apart, and it's almost too late to do anything about it!

I imagine some of you were expecting a book full of satire where I trash the crunchy lifestyle and perhaps even out myself as a—*gasp*—silky mom. (Sorry to disappoint.)

And I know there are those of you simply trying to find your way in this crazy world. You're looking for someone to help show you the best and most accessible way to live and make healthy decisions for yourself and your family.

Whatever your reason for picking it up, I hope this book was beneficial to you in some way and that it has become abundantly clear that no matter the topic, there is no one size fits all. I would hate living in a world where there was only one right way to do things. But I think we can all agree that some ways of interacting with our world are healthier than others. We can all agree that it's better for us to be outside enjoying fresh air than it is to be stuck indoors, staring at a screen. We can all agree that it's better to think about the choices you make rather than to blindly do what you're told.

Whether I've stated it outright or just made subtle hints throughout, I want you to know that you don't have to be "crunchy" to think for yourself. You aren't a conspiracy theorist if you question what big media companies tell you or if you don't believe the marketing of every company trying to make a buck off you. And that goes for your favorite influencers as well. Please, please, *please* think about and research the things I've talked about in this book for yourself. I'm not trying to be the one-stop shop for all things crunchy. Honestly? I'm just a mom who has done a lot of my own research because I'm curious about the world around me. And yes, that has led me to some conclusions in certain areas of my life, but that doesn't mean I know everything. I'm trying to do my best in a world that is trying to pull me in every direction. And I imagine it's likely the same story for you as well.

Since we're on the topic, let me briefly touch on the "conspiracy crunchy mom." She's a character I have pop up every now and then in my videos who usually says something ridiculous or out there, leaving everyone around her speechless. It usually has to do with Big Ag, Big Pharma, mind control, or chem trails. I think a lot of people out there would tell you that a path through the crunchy life must also be one filled with conspiracies and preparation for the end of the world.

And while I don't think it's a bad idea to be as prepared for disaster as possible, I also know there is a lot of money to be made in pushing conspiracies. What would we call it? Big Conspiracy?

It's very easy to be researching the negative effects of too much screen time and suddenly find yourself reading articles or watching interviews about the government's deep dark plan for population control. You then find yourself buying prepper supplies from companies that may or may not have good-quality products and certainly don't care as much about your best interests as they do lining their wallets with your hard-earned cash.

I'm not saying some of these articles and videos don't present some compelling arguments, but even if some of them are true, you have to ask yourself: Is dwelling on them going to make life better? Would you be taking steps toward macro changes or micro changes?

Just be aware of the potential traps you may find yourself in. When you do research, when you go down the rabbit holes and do the deep dives, it's easy to get sucked into the same kind of marketing that the big companies throw at you. Worst of all, and I can attest to this, it is way too easy to introduce a lot of unneeded anxiety into your life. And this is where I may be a little different from some of the crunchiest of crunchy moms: I believe that a lot of anxiety is much worse for you than the things you are anxious about.

The best approach is to look at the world around you and make small improvements where you can while not believing everything you read. Just because an article states that a study found a carcinogenic compound in America's drinking water doesn't mean you should keep yourself up at night because you let your child drink from the water fountain. Things happen; make decisions, then move on. There is no use dwelling on the past.

We've covered a lot of ground in this book, and I truly believe each topic we covered could be its own book. But I can't stress enough the importance of your relationships with both your friends and your family. If you are starting out and determined to dive into the crunchy lifestyle but you don't have the best support system, it can feel like you're bleeding in a sea full of sharks. More than likely, that's your own perception of things rather than reality. That's not to discredit your feelings. I've known my fair share of people who vehemently disagreed with how I choose to eat or the way I try to live a more natural life. But most people simply don't understand why you're doing the things you're doing, and it doesn't have to be your job to explain it to them or convert them to your way of thinking. Likely, people don't even care what you're doing—and I mean that in the best way possible. The best thing you can do is show grace to others. And if they aren't directly affecting the course you have set for yourself and your family, let them be. There might be a few jokes at your expense, or someone might feel offended that you brought your own water to an event, but in the end, *they* aren't who you're doing this for.

Before I wrap this up, I want to talk about one more thing I mentioned briefly early in the book: the whole idea of "know better, do better." While, on the surface, this principle makes sense and is technically true (if you know better, you should do better), it is certainly not an uplifting thing to say to someone when they are trying their best to navigate this world. And the problem isn't the phrase itself, even though I detest the phrase now—it's the sentiment. It's the lack of compassion and empathy that some of us let take hold of our hearts and minds when we're on a journey like this. So many of us are unsure about so many things. I would wager that most people taking steps toward a crunchier lifestyle, especially those who weren't raised in it, are doing so with the best intentions and spend half the time scared to death that they aren't doing something right.

The "know better, do better" attitude is as toxic as a cinnamon bun–scented candle (well, maybe not, but you know what I mean). It discourages others from wanting to dive deeper into a lifestyle that is good for them and their families. It makes people feel small.

If you watch a lot of my videos, then you've no doubt come across a series where I play the part of two crunchy moms who are trying to "outcrunch" each other. Yes, it is as ridiculous as it sounds. One mom is bragging about the natural fibers in her clothing, while the other mom comes back with how the frequencies of those fibers cancel one another out, thereby negating the benefits. I can't tell you how many times I've seen this kind of interaction, whether in person, in the comments section, or even in messages I receive. I'll be honest, even when I get a comment in jest on a video saying that an aspect of it wasn't quite crunchy enough (followed by "know better, do better"), I can't help but cringe inside. It's a small suppression of anger and that feeling of belittlement. I know the commentor was joking (most of the time), but the sentiment still triggers a response in me that I don't like.

Remember Amy from the beginning of the book? The one who said, "This is actually so toxic," when I gifted her a bottle of hand soap? That's what I'm talking about here. Back then, I was still learning about all this. And I'm still learning about it. Truth be told, for some people, what I know and what I implement in my life will never be enough. That's why you have to remember that your journey isn't about them. It's not about impressing others or comparing your life to someone else's. Is it not apparent by now that keeping up with the Joneses is the farthest thing from crunchy there is?

You don't need what someone else has. You shouldn't want what someone else has. They are on their journey, and you are on yours. Never forget that.

The word *crunchy* is a label—an easy way for people to identify others or themselves if their lives are following a path toward a more natural way of life. But even that is changing. When I started the Really Very Crunchy comedy account, it was a niche group with their own stereotypes. Why do you think it was so easy to come up with funny content about crunchy people? But the world is waking up to "crunchy." Or, put another way, people are starting to realize that leaning into a natural way of living makes a lot more sense than the direction we've been going for the past few decades. People are asking more questions. They are becoming informed about what's going into their food, their cosmetics, their bloodstreams.

In short, the crunchiest things you can do are think for yourself, do the best you can, and show love to your fellow human beings.

Acknowledgments

Out of a thousand things I expected to do in my life, creating a comedy channel with my husband that ended up gaining enough followers that a publisher would want me to write a book about my experiences was not one of them.

This, of course, would not have happened without my agent, Tom Dean. At the very beginning of this process, he helped me shape this book in the idea stage to make it something a publisher would consider looking at. I've never worked with someone so responsive and so excited about a project. At times I thought he was more excited about this book than I was, which is saying a lot! Tom has believed in this project from the moment it reached his desk, and I don't think I could have had a better ally in the publishing world.

However, it was his daughter, Ashleigh Pinkerton, who brought the Really Very Crunchy account to his attention. I was absolutely delighted when I found out she was going to help me with marketing and even content ideas to go along with the book launch. The two of them are an unmatched duo in their field, and I am forever blessed that they stepped into my life.

My editors, Carly Kellerman and Kim Tanner, were saints throughout the editing process. In less-skilled hands, this book likely would have been a structural mess, and you may have left it more confused than if you hadn't read it in the first place.

I would also like to thank my parents, who sacrificed time and time again to give me more opportunities than they had, for being so encouraging and supportive every step of the way, and for forgiving me of my flaws and loving me regardless.

Thank you to my husband, Jason, though I'm not sure I should thank him. He sort of got me into this mess. (I'm kidding, Love.) In all seriousness, not only was he a huge encouragement throughout the writing and editing process, but without him, I wouldn't have started Really Very Crunchy at all. Both of us love being creative, and we both love creating comedy, but Jason was insistent that we start in 2022. "It's going to be big!" he said over and over. It took him about six months to finally convince me to do it. I can say this: it was every bit as big as he foresaw and then some. Without his camerawork, editing, and genius comedic timing, you wouldn't get Really Very Crunchy videos. And without his unwavering support and encouragement, you wouldn't have this book either.

All that said, even with the support from the professionals in the industry and from my husband at home, none of this would matter without each and every one of you who has shown up for my videos. I am honored by the opportunity you have given me. I try to read every comment, I take note of every like, and I am beyond blessed to have this community that has shown me nothing but love since day one. Thank you for supporting me. Thank you for being amazing. Thank you for all the likes, the comments, and the messages. I'm grateful for every single one of you, and I hope this book is a small light in your life.

Resources

BOOKS
On Spending Time Outdoors

1000 Hours Outside: Activities to Match Screen Time with Green Time **and** *Until the Streetlights Come On: How a Return to Play Brightens Our Present and Prepares Kids for an Uncertain Future* by Ginny Yurich

Backyard and Beyond: A Guide for Discovering the Outdoors by Edward Duensing and A. B. Millmoss

Balanced and Barefoot: How Unrestricted Outdoor Play Makes for Strong, Confident, and Capable Children by Angela J. Hanscom

The Lost Art of Reading Nature's Signs: Use Outdoor Clues to Find Your Way, Predict the Weather, Locate Water, Track Animals—and Other Forgotten Skills by Tristan Gooley

On Living

The Encyclopedia of Country Living, 50th Anniversary Edition: The Original Manual for Living Off the Land and Doing It Yourself by Carla Emery

*A Healthier Home: The Room-by-Room Guide to Make Any
    Space a Little Less Toxic* by Shawna Holman
*Simply Living Well: A Guide to Creating a Natural, Low-Waste
    Home* by Julia Watkins

On Parenting

*Adventuring Together: How to Create Connections and Make
    Lasting Memories with Your Kids* by Greta Eskridge
M is for Mama: A Rebellion against Mediocre Motherhood by
    Abbie Halberstadt
*The Read-Aloud Family: Making Meaningful and Lasting
    Connections with Your Kids* by Sarah Mackenzie
*Smart Medicine for a Healthier Child: A Practical A-to-Z
    Reference to Natural and Conventional Treatments for
    Infants and Children* by Janet Zand, Robert Roundtree,
    and Rachel Walton
*The Whole-Brain Child: 12 Revolutionary Strategies to Nurture
    Your Child's Developing Mind* by Daniel J. Siegel and Tina
    Payne Bryson

MY FAVORITE SHOPS
Bedding, Clothing, and Shoes

NATURAL BEDDING

- https://birchliving.com
- https://redlandcotton.com

SUSTAINABLE CLOTHING

- https://www.etsy.com

- https://magiclinen.com
- https://pyneandsmith.com/collections/dresses
- https://www.toadandco.com

BAREFOOT SHOES

- https://us.wildling.shoes
- https://splayshoes.com
- https://www.vivobarefoot.com/us/

Cookware

CAST IRON

- https://www.lodgecastiron.com

STAINLESS STEEL PANS

- https://www.360cookware.com
- https://www.all-clad.com

Nontoxic Beauty

MAKEUP

- https://toupsandco.com
- https://www.truthgirl.com

SKINCARE

- https://www.bigwoodsorganics.com
- https://www.etsy.com/shop/PineandSageHerbals
- https://nourishyounaturally.com
- https://smithfarm1914.com

- https://toupsandco.com
- https://www.whitewoodherbarie.com

WRINKLE TAPE

- https://www.frownies.com

Water

- https://www.clearlyfiltered.com for pitcher
- https://www.greenfieldwater.com for countertop and whole home
- https://www.ispringwatersystems.com for under the sink and whole home
- https://lifestraw.com for on the go

Wellness

HERBAL TINCTURES

- https://earthley.com
- https://goldengardenflorida.com
- https://www.hawthornandhoney.com/shop

SUPPLEMENTS

- https://ancestralsupplements.com
- https://www.greenpasture.org
- https://mountainroseherbs.com

SOCIAL MEDIA ACCOUNTS

@theappalachianhomestead on Instagram and YouTube

for wisdom from ninth-generation homesteaders on
gardening, canning, and folkways
@fallondanae on Instagram for simple, nourishing food ideas
@foxmeetsbear on Instagram for outdoor exploration,
homemaking, and creating connections with your kids
@growforagecookferment on Instagram for excellent healthy
recipes
@homegrown_education on Instagram for great information
on real food for the whole family
@thehomesteadingrd on Instagram for encouraging
self-sufficiency
@the.hopewellhomestead on Instagram for accessible holistic
living
@leafandlearn on Instagram for encouragement for the home
educator
@northwoodsfolk on Instagram for nature-inspired
mothering and beautiful seasonal crafts
@nourished.lifestyle.home on Instagram for simple food
swaps and healthy meal ideas
@tessaromero_on Instagram for helpful mindset shifts that
will change your perspective on mothering

References

Chapter 4: The Basic Needs (Part 1)

1. Fred Rogers, "Remembering Mr. Rogers (1994/1997)," interview by Charlie Rose, aired September 20, 1994, on PBS, video shared by Charlie Rose, February 27, 2016, on YouTube, 2:24,. www.youtube.com/watch?v=djoyd46TVVc&ab_channel=CharlieRose.

2. Dr. Seuss, *How the Grinch Stole Christmas* (New York: Random House Children's Books, 1985), 10.

3. "Initial List of Hazardous Air Pollutants with Modifications," United States Environmental Protection Agency, last updated December 19, 2022, www.epa.gov/haps/initial-list-hazardous-air-pollutants-modifications.

4. "What Are Hazardous Air Pollutants?," United States Environmental Protection Agency, last updated December 19, 2022, www.epa.gov/haps/what-are-hazardous-air-pollutants.

5. Ralph Waldo Emerson, "Merlin's Song," in *Poems: Household Edition* (Boston: Houghton, Mifflin and Company, 1904), 219, en.wikisource.org/wiki/Poems_(Emerson,_Household_Edition,_1904)/Merlin%27s_Song.

6. "The Inside Story: A Guide to Indoor Air Quality," United States Environmental Protection Agency, last updated June 22, 2023, www.epa.gov/indoor-air-quality-iaq/inside-story-guide -indoor-air-quality.

7. Mei Chen et al., "Residential Exposure to Pesticide during Childhood and Childhood Cancers: A Meta-analysis," *Pediatrics* 136, no. 4 (October 2015): https://doi.org/10.1542 /peds.2015-0006.

8. Ryan Felton, Lisa Gill, and Lewis Kendall, "We Sampled Tap Water across the US—and Found Arsenic, Lead and Toxic Chemicals," *Guardian*, March 31, 2021, www.theguardian .com/us-news/2021/mar/31/americas-tap-water-samples -forever-chemicals.

9. Felton, Gill, and Kendall, "We Sampled Tap Water."

10. Kanwal Rehman, Fiza Fatima, Iqra Waheed, and Muhammad Sajid Hamid Akash, "Prevalence of Exposure of Heavy Metals and Their Impact on Health Consequences," *Journal of Cellular Biochemistry* 119, no. 1 (January 2018): 157–84, https://www .doi.org/10.1002/jcb.26234.

11. World Health Organization, "Microplastics in Drinking-Water," August 28, 2019, https://www.who.int/publications/i /item/9789241516198.

12. Amanda MacMillan, "Safe Drinking Water," National Resources Defense Council, May 2, 2017, https://www.nrdc .org/stories/whats-your-drinking-water.

13. Nidhi Subbaraman, "These Five Brands of Dental Floss May Expose People To Harmful Chemicals, Study Finds," BuzzFeed News, January 9, 2019, https://www.buzzfeednews .com/article/nidhisubbaraman/oral-b-pfas-dental-floss.

14. Felipe Mendes Delpino et al., "Ultra-processed Food and Risk of Type 2 Diabetes: A Systematic Review and Meta-analysis of Longitudinal Studies," *International Journal of Epidemiology* 51, no. 4 (August 2022): https://doi.org/10.1093/ije/dyab247.

15. "Ultra-processed Foods Linked to Poor Heart Health," Harvard Health Publishing, September 1, 2019, https://www.health .harvard.edu/heart-health/ultra-processed-foods-linked-to-poor -heart-health.

16. Laure Schnabel, Camille Buscail, Jean-Marc Sabate, Michel Bouchoucha, Emmanuelle Kesse-Guyot, Benjamin Allès, Mathilde Touvier, Carlos A. Monteiro, Serge Hercberg, Robert Benamouzig, Chantal Julia, "Association Between Ultra-processed Food Consumption and Functional Gastrointestinal Disorders: Results from the French NutriNet-Santé Cohort," *American Journal of Gastroenterology* 113, no. 8 (August 2018): 1217–228, https://doi.org10.1038/s41395-018-0137-1.

17. Thibault Fiolet et al., "Consumption of Ultra-processed Foods and Cancer Risk: Results from NutriNet-Santé Prospective Cohort," *BMJ* 360 (February 2018): https://doi.org/10.1136/bmj.k322.

18. Ed Ergenzinger, "Adverse Effects of Ultra-processed Foods on Mental Health," *Psychology Today*, September 12, 2022, https://www.psychologytoday.com/us/blog/night-sweats-and -delusions-grandeur/202209/adverse-effects-ultra-processed -foods-mental-health.

19. A. Shafik, I. H. Ibrahim, and E. M. El-Sayed, "Effect of Different Types of Textile Fabric on Spermatogenesis I. Electrostatic Potentials Generated on Surface of Human Scrotum by Wearing Different Types of Fabric," *Andrologia* 24, no. 3 (May–June 1992): https://doi.org/10.1111/j.1439-0272 .1992.tb02628.x.

20. Caitlin O'Kane, "Children's Clothing Sets Sold at TJ Maxx, Amazon and Other Retailers Have Been Recalled for Lead Paint," CBS News, December 1, 2022, https://www.cbsnews .com/news/childrens-clothing-recall-lead-paint-bentex-sold-a -tjmaxx-amazon-disney-characters-screen-print-designs-refund/.

21. Rashmila Maiti, "Fast Fashion and Its Environmental Impact," Earth.org, May 21, 2023, https://earth.org/fast-fashions -detrimental-effect-on-the-environment/.

22. Mark Anthony Browne et al., "Accumulation of Microplastic on Shorelines Worldwide: Sources and Sinks," *Environmental Science and Technology* 45, no. 21 (September 2011): https:// doi.org/10.1021/es201811s.

23. Olivia Lai, "7 Fast Fashion Companies Responsible for Environmental Pollution in 2022," Earth.org, October 15, 2022, https://earth.org/fast-fashion-companies/.

Chapter 5: The Basic Needs (Part 2)

1. Andy R. Eugene and Jolanta Masiak, "The Neuroprotective Aspects of Sleep," *MEDtube Science* 3, no. 1 (March 2015): www.ncbi.nlm.nih.gov/pmc/articles/PMC4651462/.

2. Masahiro Banno et al., "Exercise Can Improve Sleep Quality: A Systematic Review and Meta-analysis," *PeerJ* 6 (July 2018): https://doi.org/10.7717/peerj.5172.

3. Young Ran Kim et al., "Health Consequences of Exposure to Brominated Flame Retardants: A Systematic Review," *Chemosphere* 106 (July 2014): https://doi.org/10.1016/j .chemosphere.2013.12.064.

4. "Formaldehyde and Cancer Risk," National Cancer Institute, last reviewed June 10, 2011, https://www.cancer.gov/about

-cancer/causes-prevention/risk/substances/formaldehyde
/formaldehyde-fact-sheet.

5. Tasha Stoiber, "What Are Parabens, And Why Don't They Belong in Cosmetics?," Environmental Working Group, April 9, 2019, https://www.ewg.org/what-are-parabens.

6. "What Are the Health Effects of PFAS," Agency for Toxic Substances and Disease Registry, last reviewed November 1, 2022, https://www.atsdr.cdc.gov/pfas/health-effects/index.html.

7. Rachel Shaffer, "The Chemicals Called PFCs Are Everywhere, and That's a Problem," Environmental Defense Fund, April 30, 2013, https://www.edf.org/blog/2013/04/30/chemicals-called -pfcs-are-everywhere-and-thats-problem.

8. Kyle L. Alford and Naresh Kumar, "Pulmonary Health Effects of Indoor Volatile Organic Compounds—a Meta-analysis," *International Journal of Environmental Research and Public Health* 18, no. 4 (February 2021): https://doi.org/10.3390 /ijerph18041578.

Chapter 6: When Your Family Isn't Crunchy

1. "Asbestos Disease Awareness Organization Releases Findings That Reveal Evidence of Asbestos in Everyday Products," ADAO, November 28, 2007, https://www.ewg.org/sites /default/files/ADAOasbestos_20071204.pdf.

2. Dale Carnegie, *How to Win Friends and Influence People* (1936; repr., New Delhi, India: Srishti, 2020), 131.

3. Sarah Kobylewski and Michael F. Jacobson, "Toxicology of Food Dyes," *International Journal of Occupational and Environmental Health* 18, no. 3 (2012): https://doi.org/10.1179 /1077352512Z.00000000034.

Chapter 8: Making Crunchy Kids

1. Nicole E. Marshall, Barbara Abrams, Linda A. Barbour, Patrick Catalano, Parul Christian, Jacob E. Friedman, William W. Hay Jr., Teri L. Hernandez, Nancy F. Krebs, Emily Oken, Jonathan Q. Purnell, James M. Roberts, Hora Soltani, Jacqueline Wallace, Kent L. Thornburg, "The Importance of Nutrition in Pregnancy and Lactation: Lifelong Consequences," *American Journal of Obstetrics and Gynecology* 226, no. 5 (May 2022): 607–32, https://doi.org/10.1016/j.ajog.2021.12.035.

2. Sarah Cusick and Michael K. Georgieff, "The First 1,000 Days of Life: The Brain's Window of Opportunity," Unicef, April 12, 2013, https://www.unicef-irc.org/article/958-the-first-1000-days-of-life-the-brains-window-of-opportunity.html.

3. Philippians 4:6.

4. Alexandra Lautarescu, Michael C. Craig, and Vivette Glover, "Prenatal Stress: Effects on Fetal and Child Brain Development," *International Review of Neurobiology* 150 (March 2020): https://doi.org/10.1016/bs.irn.2019.11.002.

5. Sarah J. Buckley, *Hormonal Physiology of Childbearing: Evidence and Implications for Women, Babies, and Maternity Care* (Washington, DC: Childbirth Connection Programs, National Partnership for Women & Families, January 2015).

6. "Delayed Umbilical Cord Clamping after Birth. ACOG Committee Opinion No. 814," American College of Obstetricians and Gynecologists, *Obstetrics and Gynecology* 136, no. 6 (December 2020): e100–e106, https://doi.org/10.1097/AOG.0000000000004167.

7. Maria G. Dominguez-Bello et al., "Partial Restoration of the Microbiota of Cesarean-Born Infants via Vaginal Microbial

Transfer," *Nature Medicine* 22 (March 2016): https://doi.org /10.1038/nm.4039.

8. Emily R. Dodwell, "Babywearing Is Healthy, If Done the Right Way," Hospital for Special Surgery, April 2, 2021, www.hss .edu/article_babywearing.asp.

9. Giulia Nuzzi, Maria Elisa Di Cicco, and Diego Giampietro Peroni, "Breastfeeding and Allergic Diseases: What's New?," *Children* 8, no. 5 (April 2021): https://doi.org/10.3390 /children8050330.

10. Jae Eun Shim, Juhee Kim, and Rose Ann Mathai, "Associations of Infant Feeding Practices and Picky Eating Behaviors of Preschool Children," *Journal of the Academy of Nutrition and Dietetics* 111, no. 9 (September 2011): 1363–68, https://doi .org/10.1016/j.jada.2011.06.410.

11. World Health Organization, *Q&A on Glyphosate* (Lyon, France: International Agency for Research on Cancer, March 2016), 1, www.iarc.who.int/wp-content/uploads/2018/11 /QA_Glyphosate.pdf.

12. "Get the Facts: Added Sugars," Centers for Disease Control and Prevention, last updated November 28, 2021, https:// www.cdc.gov/nutrition/data-statistics/added-sugars.html.

13. Trisha Korioth, "Added Sugar in Kids' Diets: How Much Is Too Much?," American Academy of Pediatrics, March 25, 2019, https://publications.aap.org/aapnews/news/7331/Added-sugar-in -kids-diets-How-much-is-too-much?autologinchec=redirected.

14. Karen Le Billon, *French Kids Eat Everything: How Our Family Moved to France, Cured Picky Eating, Banned Snacking, and Discovered 10 Simple Rules for Raising Happy, Healthy Eaters* (New York: William Morrow, 2012), 111.

15. Nneka Leiba and Sydney Swanson, "EWG's Healthy Living: Guide to Safer Diapers," Environmental Working Group, December 10, 2020, https://www.ewg.org/research/diaper -guide.

16. Kenneth R. Ginsburg, Committee on Communications, and Committee on Psychosocial Aspects of Child and Family Health, "The Importance of Play in Promoting Healthy Child Development and Maintaining Strong Parent-Child Bonds," *Pediatrics* 119, no. 1 (January 2007): 2006–697, https://doi .org/10.1542/peds.

17. Angela J. Hanscom, *Balanced and Barefoot: How Unrestricted Outdoor Play Makes for Strong, Confident, and Capable Children* (Oakland, CA: New Harbinger, 2016), 167.

Chapter 9: A Crunchy Home Requires Sunshine

1. "Frequently Asked Questions," Mountain Lion Foundation, accessed September 14, 2023, mountainlion.org/about -mountain-lions/frequently-asked-questions/.

2. Mathew P. White et al., "Spending at Least 120 Minutes a Week in Nature Is Associated with Good Health and Wellbeing," *Scientific Reports* 9 (June 2019): https://doi.org/10.1038/s41598 -019-44097-3.

3. Bruce Goldman, "Addictive Potential of Social Media, Explained," Stanford Medicine, October 29, 2011, https:// scopeblog.stanford.edu/2021/10/29/addictive-potential-of -social-media-explained/.

4. "Screen Time vs. Lean Time," Centers for Disease Control and Prevention, last reviewed January 29, 2018, https://www.cdc .gov/nccdphp/dnpao/multimedia/infographics/getmoving.html.

5. John S. Hutton et al., "Associations between Screen-Based Media Use and Brain White Matter Integrity in Preschool-Aged Children," *JAMA Pediatrics* 174, no. 1 (2020): https://doi.org/10.1001/jamapediatrics.2019.3869.

6. Sandee LaMotte, "MRIs Show Screen Time Linked to Lower Brain Development in Preschoolers," CNN, November 4, 2019, www.cnn.com/2019/11/04/health/screen-time-lower-brain-development-preschoolers-wellness/index.html.

7. Danette Glassy and Pooja Tandon, "Playing Outside: Why It's Important for Kids," HealthyChildren.org, American Academy of Pediatrics, last updated April 19, 2023, www.healthychildren.org/English/family-life/power-of-play/Pages/playing-outside-why-its-important-for-kids.aspx.

8. Hanmin Wang et al., "Vitamin D and Chronic Diseases," *Aging and Disease* 8, no. 3 (June 2017): https://doi.org/10.14336/AD.2016.1021.

9. Kirsten Weir, "Nurtured by Nature," *Monitor on Psychology* 51, no. 3 (April–May 2020): www.apa.org/monitor/2020/04/nurtured-nature. Weir cites Kristine Engemann et al., "Residential Green Space in Childhood Is Associated with Lower Risk of Psychiatric Disorders from Adolescence into Adulthood," *PNAS* 116, no. 11 (February 2019): https://doi.org/10.1073/pnas.1807504116.

10. James Oschman, Gaetan Chevalier, and Richard Brown, "The Effects of Grounding (Earthing) on Inflammation, the Immune Response, Wound Healing, and Prevention and Treatment of Chronic Inflammatory and Autoimmune Diseases," *Journal of Inflammation Research* 8 (March 2015): https://doi.org/10.2147/JIR.S69656.

11. Carly Rose (@rewildcarlyrose), "Humans are not meant to wake up in a box…" Instagram, September 12, 2022, https://www.instagram.com/reel/CibQFfAuFvM/.

12. "1000 Hours Outside—Join the Challenge," 1000 Hours Outside (website), accessed September 14, 2023, www.1000hoursoutside.com/blog/1000-hours-outside -2020-challenge.

Chapter 10: Beauty Is in the Eye of the Beholder

1. Thomas J. Walker and Steve H. Dayan, "Comparison and Overview of Currently Available Neurotoxins," *Journal of Clinical and Aesthetic Dermatology* 7, no. 2 (February 2014): 31–39, https://pubmed.ncbi.nlm.nih.gov/24587850/.

2. Robin Givhan, "Dangerous Beauty," *Washington Post*, October 18, 2022, www.washingtonpost.com/nation /2022/10/18/dangerous-beauty/.

3. Scott Faber, "The Toxic Twelve Chemicals and Contaminants in Cosmetics," Environmental Working Group, May 5, 2020, www.ewg.org/the-toxic-twelve-chemicals-and-contaminants -in-cosmetics.

4. "Valisure Detects High Levels of Benzene in Several Dry Shampoo Products and Requests FDA Actions," Valisure, November 1, 2022, www.valisure.com/valisure-newsroom /valisure-detects-benzene-in-dry-shampoo.

Chapter 11: Don't Waste Your Life

1. Eleanor Evins, "Disposable Menstrual Products: Impact and Alternatives," Candor Health Education, accessed October 18, 2023, https://candorhealthed.org/disposable-menstrual -products-impact-and-alternatives/.

Chapter 13: Crunchy Self-Care

1. Ashish Sharma, Vishal Madaan, and Frederick D. Petty, "Exercise for Mental Health," letter to the editor, *Primary Care Companion Journal of Clinical Psychiatry* 8, no. 2 (2006): 106, https://doi.org/10.4088/pcc.v08n0208a.

Chapter 14: Beyond Crunchy

1. Mohd Razali Salleh, "Life Event, Stress and Illness," *Malaysian Journal of Medical Sciences* 15, no. 4 (October 2008): www.ncbi.nlm.nih.gov/pmc/articles/PMC3341916/.

2. "Can Expressing Gratitude Improve Your Mental, Physical Health?," Mayo Clinic Health System, December 6, 2022, https://www.mayoclinichealthsystem.org/hometown-health /speaking-of-health/can-expressing-gratitude-improve-health.

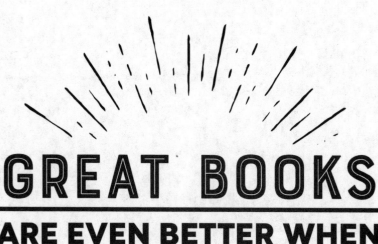